Children of Incarcerated Parents

This book highlights the myriad factors that can impact the children of incarcerated parents. It is no secret that the United States continues to be the leading nation for the incarceration of men and women, and this large prison population includes approximately 120,000 incarcerated mothers and 1.1 million incarcerated fathers. Incarceration of a parent is recognized as an "adverse childhood experience," an acute or chronic situation that for most people is stressful and potentially traumatic. Children of incarcerated parents may experience other adverse childhood experiences such as poverty, homelessness, parental substance abuse and other mental health problems, and family violence. The chapters in this book document some of the challenges as well as some promising ways that can help parents and families begin to meet these challenges. It is our hope that the compendium of chapters presented in this book will be a resource for practitioners, policy makers, educators, researchers, and advocates in their work to ensure that the children of incarcerated parents, their caregivers, and their mothers and fathers are provided the support they need to address the challenges they face during and after parental incarceration.

This book was originally published as a special issue of *Smith College Studies in Social Work*.

Marian S. Harris is a Professor of Social Work and child welfare researcher in the Social Work and Criminal Justice Program at the University of Washington Tacoma, USA.

J. Mark Eddy is a senior research scientist and licensed psychologist with the Family Translational Research Group at New York University, USA.

Children of Incarcerated Parents
Challenges and Promise

Edited by
Marian S. Harris and J. Mark Eddy

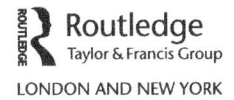

Routledge
Taylor & Francis Group

LONDON AND NEW YORK

First published 2018
by Routledge
2 Park Square, Milton Park, Abingdon, Oxon, OX14 4RN, UK

and by Routledge
711 Third Avenue, New York, NY 10017, USA

Routledge is an imprint of the Taylor & Francis Group, an informa business

© 2018 Taylor & Francis

All rights reserved. No part of this book may be reprinted or reproduced or utilised in any form or by any electronic, mechanical, or other means, now known or hereafter invented, including photocopying and recording, or in any information storage or retrieval system, without permission in writing from the publishers.

Trademark notice: Product or corporate names may be trademarks or registered trademarks, and are used only for identification and explanation without intent to infringe.

British Library Cataloguing in Publication Data
A catalogue record for this book is available from the British Library

ISBN13: 978-1-138-57157-0

Typeset in MinionPro
by diacriTech, Chennai

Publisher's Note
The publisher accepts responsibility for any inconsistencies that may have arisen during the conversion of this book from journal articles to book chapters, namely the possible inclusion of journal terminology.

Disclaimer
Every effort has been made to contact copyright holders for their permission to reprint material in this book. The publishers would be grateful to hear from any copyright holder who is not here acknowledged and will undertake to rectify any errors or omissions in future editions of this book.

Contents

Citation Information vii
Notes on Contributors ix

Introduction 1
Marian S. Harris and J. Mark Eddy

1 Early Relational Health: Infants' Experiences Living with Their
  Incarcerated Mothers 4
  Marie-Celeste Condon

2 Incarcerated Mothers: Trauma and Attachment Issues 25
  Marian S. Harris

3 Substance Use among Youth with Currently and Formerly
  Incarcerated Parents 42
  Laurel Davis and Rebecca J. Shlafer

4 Variations in the Life Histories of Incarcerated Parents by Race
  and Ethnicity: Implications for Service Provision 58
  Keva M. Miller, J. Mark Eddy, Sharon Borja, and Sarah R. Lazzari

5 A Statewide Parenting Alternative Sentencing Program: Description
  and Preliminary Outcomes 77
  Chyla M. Aguiar and Susan Leavell

6 The Moderating Effect of Living with a Child Before Incarceration on Postrelease
  Outcomes Related to a Prison-Based Parent Management
  Training Program 93
  Bert O. Burraston and J. Mark Eddy

7 Building a Tailored, Multilevel Prevention Strategy to Support Children
  and Families Affected by Parental Incarceration 111
  Jean Kjellstrand

Index 129

Citation Information

The chapters in this book were originally published in *Smith College Studies in Social Work*, volume 87, issue 1 (January–March 2017). When citing this material, please use the original page numbering for each article, as follows:

Introduction
Guest Editorial
Marian S. Harris and J. Mark Eddy
Smith College Studies in Social Work, volume 87, issue 1 (January–March 2017)
pp. 2–4

Chapter 1
Early Relational Health: Infants' Experiences Living with Their Incarcerated Mothers
Marie-Celeste Condon
Smith College Studies in Social Work, volume 87, issue 1 (January–March 2017)
pp. 5–25

Chapter 2
Incarcerated Mothers: Trauma and Attachment Issues
Marian S. Harris
Smith College Studies in Social Work, volume 87, issue 1 (January–March 2017)
pp. 26–42

Chapter 3
Substance Use among Youth with Currently and Formerly Incarcerated Parents
Laurel Davis and Rebecca J. Shlafer
Smith College Studies in Social Work, volume 87, issue 1 (January–March 2017)
pp. 43–58

Chapter 4
Variations in the Life Histories of Incarcerated Parents by Race and Ethnicity: Implications for Service Provision
Keva M. Miller, J. Mark Eddy, Sharon Borja, and Sarah R. Lazzari
Smith College Studies in Social Work, volume 87, issue 1 (January–March 2017)
pp. 59–77

CITATION INFORMATION

Chapter 5
A Statewide Parenting Alternative Sentencing Program: Description and Preliminary Outcomes
Chyla M. Aguiar and Susan Leavell
Smith College Studies in Social Work, volume 87, issue 1 (January–March 2017)
pp. 78–93

Chapter 6
The Moderating Effect of Living with a Child Before Incarceration on Postrelease Outcomes Related to a Prison-Based Parent Management Training Program
Bert O. Burraston and J. Mark Eddy
Smith College Studies in Social Work, volume 87, issue 1 (January–March 2017)
pp. 94–111

Chapter 7
Building a Tailored, Multilevel Prevention Strategy to Support Children and Families Affected by Parental Incarceration
Jean Kjellstrand
Smith College Studies in Social Work, volume 87, issue 1 (January–March 2017)
pp. 112–129

For any permission-related enquiries please visit:
http://www.tandfonline.com/page/help/permissions

Notes on Contributors

Chyla M. Aguiar, MA, is a research associate at the Washington State Institute for Criminal Justice in Spokane, Washington, and a doctoral candidate in criminal justice and criminology at Washington State University, USA. Her research interests include international continuity, reentry and alternatives to incarceration initiatives, evidence-based practices, and evaluation research.

Sharon Borja, MSW, is a PhD candidate at the School of Social Work, University of Washington, USA. Her research focuses on child well-being, parent mental health, and the long-reaching influence of life course and intergenerational adversity. She is especially interested in the developmental and social context of adversity accumulation, particularly among families of color who are often at the intersection of racial disparities and multiple systems involvement.

Bert O. Burraston, PhD, is an Assistant Professor and the graduate coordinator in the Department of Criminology and Criminal Justice at the University of Memphis, USA. His research focuses on program evaluation, offender reentry, child and adolescent development, poverty, and advanced statistics.

Marie-Celeste Condon, PhD, is an infant and early childhood mental health consultant in private practice and she is a Level IV Mentor in Infant Mental Health. Her research focuses on early relational health, and understanding and describing children's experiences during the first 1000 days of life.

Laurel Davis, PhD, is a Postdoctoral Fellow in the Division of General Pediatrics and Adolescent Health at the University of Minnesota-Twin Cities. Her research focuses on the prevention of social, emotional, and behavioral problems in young people facing adversity.

J. Mark Eddy is a Senior Research Scientist and licensed psychologist with the Family Translational Research Group at New York University, USA.

Marian S. Harris is a Professor of Social Work in the Social Work and Criminal Justice Program at the University of Washington Tacoma, USA.

Jean Kjellstrand, PhD, is an Assistant Research Professor at the Center for Equity Promotion within the College of Education at the University of Oregon, USA. She is also an Assistant Research Scientist at Columbia University in New York, USA. Her research examines the role of key individual, family, and community factors on the development of children with criminal justice-involved parents.

NOTES ON CONTRIBUTORS

Sarah R. Lazzari, MS, is a PhD candidate in the School of Social Work at Portland State University, USA. Her research interests are focused on how an individual's community/family support networks are affected by periods of incarceration.

Susan Leavell is a program administrator for the Washington State Department of Corrections (DOC), USA; she directs parent alternative sentencing programs. She has worked in corrections and law enforcement for 30 years and has built a career in doing reentry work with offenders leaving prison. She works closely with community organizations to provide opportunities for offenders in education, skills building, employment, and other needs.

Keva M. Miller, PhD, is Associate Dean for Academic Affairs and Associate Professor at Portland State University, USA. Her research focuses on children of criminal justice-involved parents, incarcerated parents, justice-involved parents, racial disproportionality and disparity in criminal justice and child welfare systems, social injustices and inequities, and African Americans.

Rebecca J. Shlafer, PhD, MPH, is an Assistant Professor in the Division of General Pediatrics and Adolescent Health. Her research focuses on understanding the developmental outcomes of children and families in the criminal justice system. She is particularly interested in children with incarcerated parents, as well as the programs and policies that impact families affected by incarceration.

Introduction

This special issue features a broad continuum of articles that highlight the myriad factors that can impact the children of incarcerated parents. It is no secret that the United States continues to be the leading nation for the incarceration of men and women in the world. Many of these people are parents. It was recently estimated that in prisons in the United States, on any given day, more than 120,000 incarcerated mothers and 1.1 million incarcerated fathers are the parents of minor children under 10 years of age (Glaze & Maruschak, 2011). Many more children have parents who are incarcerated in jails or were incarcerated in jails or prisons in the past.

Incarceration of a parent is recognized as an "adverse childhood experience," an acute or a chronic situation that for most people is stressful and may be traumatic. Adverse childhood experiences not only are related to negative consequences in children but also have been demonstrated to significantly affect an individual's likelihood of experiencing a variety of negative experiences during adulthood, including additional adverse events (Fetelli et al., 1998). Children of incarcerated parents may experience other adverse childhood experiences, such as poverty, homelessness, parental substance abuse and other mental health problems, and family violence. For these and a host of other reasons, parental incarceration presents significant challenges for children, families, and communities (Eddy & Poehlmann, 2010; Travis & Waul, 2003).

The seven articles in this volume document some of these challenges as well as some promising ways that can help parents and families begin to meet these challenges. Articles were chosen to illustrate the range of issues very much in need of further study. These include going beyond the simple, and profoundly troubling, recognition that there are racial and ethnic disparities within the criminal justice system and examining the usefulness of multilevel solutions for meaningfully changing this situation; investigating the impact of a developmental approach to clinical and preventive interventions for incarcerated parents, their families, and their children; considering the use of multiple points of intervention as a parent moves through arrest, jail, trial, prison, and community corrections; and using rigorous scientific research designs to study these and other issues not just once, but multiple times, because a fundamental requirement of the scientific process is the replication of results.

This volume begins with a report of a phenomenological study by Marie-Celeste Condon on the early relational experiences of infants of incarcerated mothers. In a few prisons in the United States, mothers and their infants are allowed to live together. The longest running program was established in 1901 at the Bedford Hills Correctional Facility for Women in New York State. Condon describes the experiences of infants living with their incarcerated mothers in a relationship-focused residential parenting program in a women's correctional facility. Through insights gained from repeated observations in multiple settings over an extended period of time, Condon provides the reader glimpses into the inner worlds of infants and their relationships with their primary caretakers.

This work is complemented and extended by a report by Marian S. Harris on the more typical situation: parent–child separation during incarceration. Participants were women residing in a minimum security women's correctional facility who were involved with the child welfare system. Through in person interviews, unresolved issues of trauma and disrupted attachments are explored. The impacts of parental incarceration on children are then examined by Laurel Davis and Rebecca J. Shlafer. Using data collected from students attending public schools throughout an entire state, the relations between past and current parental incarceration and the early use and misuse of alcohol, tobacco, marijuana, and prescription drugs are explored. Given the high use of substances by many incarcerated mothers and fathers during the time they committed the crimes that led to their incarceration, this particular outcome is of keen interest. Substance use may be an important part of the "intergenerational transmission" of crime and the experience of punishment. Keva M. Miller, J. Mark Eddy, Sharon Borja, and Sarah R. Lazzari then explore relations between race and ethnicity and the life histories of incarcerated mothers and fathers. Few such studies have been conducted, and identifying whether any differences exist across demographic subgroups might assist in the design of a more effective service array.

The volume then turns from documenting challenges to examining the promise of programs designed to address challenges. Of particular interest are programs that recognize, build on, and extend the strengths of an incarcerated parent and his or her family and then go on to provide ongoing support. An understudied mode in these regards is alternative sentencing for parents. These pioneering programs attempt to strengthen family bonds, encourage the development and use of prosocial skills among parents, and use a positive problem-solving approach to community corrections. At their essence, alternative sentencing programs have the potential to not only hold individuals accountable but also keep individuals connected to the fabric of society—with their families, with their neighborhoods, and with their jobs. Chyla M. Aguiar and Susan Leavell discuss two alternative sentencing alternatives for parents with minor children that are currently used throughout a state and then present preliminary outcome findings.

Some form of parent education is often a part of programming for incarcerated parents, including alternative sentencing programs. Most of the discussion in the field on parent education has focused on programs delivered in prisons. Bert O. Burraston and J. Mark Eddy examine the moderation of outcomes in a randomized controlled trial of a prison-based parent management training program. Rigorous studies of parenting programs for incarcerated parents are few, and the moderation or mediation of effects in these studies are rarely examined. In the concluding piece in this volume, Jean Kjellstrand provides an overview of the plethora of programs that have been proposed for the children of incarcerated parents and discusses how these might be put together in a way that addresses the needs of individual children, their incarcerated parents, and their families.

It is our hope that the compendium of articles presented in this special issue will be a resource for practitioners, policy makers, educators, researchers, and advocates in their work to ensure that the children of incarcerated parents, their caregivers, and their mothers and fathers are provided the support they need to address the challenges they face during and after parental incarceration and to thrive in their homes and their communities.

Marian S. Harris, PhD, LICSW, ACSW

J. Mark Eddy, PhD

References

Eddy, J. M., & Poehlmann, J. (Eds.). (2010). *Children of incarcerated parents: A handbook for researchers and practitioners*. Washington, DC: Urban Institute Press.

Fetelli, V. J., Anda, R. F., Nordenberg, D., Williamson, D., Spitz, A. M., Edwards, V. ... Marks, J. S. (1998). Relationship of childhood abuse and household dysfunction to many of the leading causes of death in adults: The adverse childhood experiences (ACE) study. *American Journal of Preventive Medicine, 14*(4), 245–258. doi:10.1016/S0749-3797(98)00017-8

Glaze, L. E., & Maruschak, L. M. (2011). *Parents in prison and their minor children*. Washington, DC: Bureau of Justice Statistics.

Travis, J., & Waul, M. (Eds.). (2003). *Prisoners once removed: The impact of incarceration and reentry on children, families, and communities*. Washington, DC: Urban Institute Press.

Early Relational Health: Infants' Experiences Living with Their Incarcerated Mothers

Marie-Celeste Condon, PhD

ABSTRACT

Little is known about the experiences and inner worlds of infants who live with their parents in prison-based residential programs. Infant observation and qualitative methods were used to study the experiences of seventeen infants living with their incarcerated mothers in a women's correctional facility. Glimpses into their inner worlds provide insights into factors that hearten and hinder early relational health. Practitioners and parents can use a relational health approach to recognize and cultivate budding capacities in infant-parent relationships. The researcher discusses the usefulness and relevance of infants' accounts for communities of practice and research.

Many infants in the United States have incarcerated parents (Pattillo, Weiman, & Western, 2004; Rebecca Project, 2010; Villanueva, 2009) and are at risk for poor social outcomes, partially as a result of disrupted attachment relationships (Cassidy, Poehlmann, & Shaver, 2010; Kjellstrand & Eddy, 2011; Lange, 2008; Myerson, Otteson, & Ryba, 2010). Although rigorous studies are few, parent–child relationship-focused interventions conducted in jails, as part of prison-based residential parenting programs, and during community-based alternative sentencing programs appear to positively affect parenting, attachments and infant and child behavior (Baradon, Fonagy, Bland, Lenard, & Sleed, 2008; Byrne, Goshin, & Joestl, 2010; Cassidy et al., 2010, 2010; Condon, Carver, Crawley, Freeman, & Van Cleave, 2010; Eddy et al., 2008; Fearn & Parker, 2004; Goshin & Byrne, 2009; Sleed, Baradon, & Fonagy, 2013). As more such programs are developed and tested, a body of research is accruing that provides insight into life stressors and felt experiences of incarcerated parents that can be used to help shape content and process, at least in regard to parents (Berry & Eigenberg, 2003; Borelli, Goshin, Joestl, Clark, & Byrne, 2010; Borja, Nurius, & Eddy, 2015; Fritz & Whitecare, 2016; Harris, 2014; Kjellstrand & Eddy, 2011; Whaley, Moe, Eddy, & Dougherty, 2008). Little is known about the experiences and inner worlds of infants and young children of incarcerated parents (Condon Weisenburg, 2011).

What can infants communicate to us about their experiences? Quite a bit, it turns out. Attachment theory is the frame of reference for this study. Researchers working within that frame have pioneered the use of techniques to help in understanding infants' experiences. In the 1940s, John Bowlby and Esther Bick developed a clinical technique called infant observation. It has long been used to hone clinicians' understanding of the situated meanings of infant behaviors, infants' inner worlds, and the psychodynamics of infant–parent relationships (Bick, 1964/1987; Waddell, 2013). Work by scholars, practitioners, and researchers that is particularly relevant to the work conducted in this study include descriptions of attachment behavior (Ainsworth, Blehar, Waters, & Wall, 1978; Cassidy, 1999; Powell, Cooper, Hoffman, & Marvin, 2013; Spieker, Nelson, & Condon, 2011), how attachment relationships develop (Brazelton & Cramer, 1990; Cassidy, 1999; Crittenden, 2008; Karen, 1994; Stern, 1985, 1990, 1995, 2002), parents' states of mind (Crittenden & Landini, 2011; Powell, Cooper, Hoffman, & Marvin, 2007; Shlafer & Poehlman, 2010; Shlafer, Raby, Laler, Hesemeyer, & Roisman, 2015; Stern, 1995), factors that influence relationship development (Belsky, 1999; Berlin, Ziv, Amaya-Jackson, & Greenberg, 2005; Crittenden & Claussen, 2000; Fraiberg, Adelson, & Shapiro, 1975; Howes, 1999; McHale, 2007; Sameroff, McDonough, & Rosenblum, 2004; Shlafer, Raby, Laler, Hesemeyer, & Roisman, 2015), the inner worlds of infants (Lieberman, 1993), infants' attachment models (Johnson, Dweck, & Chen, 2007), infant mental health (Zeanah, 2009), and infant mental health interventions (Cicchetti, Rogosch, & Toth, 2006; Katz, Lederman, & Osofsky, 2011; Lieberman & Amaya-Jackson, 2005; Lombardi & Bogle, 2004; Makariev & Shaver, 2010; Osofsky, 2004). Collectively, this body of work influences policy as well as practice (Jones Harden, 2007) and the development of new research paradigms and tools. A relational health paradigm that has proved useful in describing trends in infant–parent interactions over time (Condon, Willis, & Eddy, 2016) also proved useful in understanding the relationship experiences of infants in the RPP.

Early relational health is a function of overarching emotional tone and mutual competencies that can be observed during interactions between an infant or toddler and a parent or caregiver. The fundamental concept is mutuality, meaning relational health is not the sum of individuals' skill sets. Relational health is a categorical description of a relationship between a young child and adult. When relational health is robust the following mutual capacities develop during the first 1000 days of life: engagement; enjoyment; responsiveness; attention; pacing; initiation; imitation; cooperation; mutual ability to recognize the other person's affect, develop a shared goal, and respond to challenges; and mutual engagement in pretend play, complex communication and language, and mutual ability to build bridges between ideas (Condon et al., 2016). In relationships with positive overarching emotional tone, the parent and child develop and practice mutual capacities that sustain and strengthen their connection with one another almost effortlessly. Positive overarching emotion does not mean there are never missteps, ruptures, and upsets, only that a sense of warm connection predominates, and that ruptures can be readily repaired. Over time, these dyads develop and sustain secure, mutually heartening relationships. When overarching emotion in interactions is less than positive or negative, efforts to connect are constricted or stymied. Negative overarching emotion does not mean there is never laughter, only that missteps, ruptures, and upsets occur frequently, and are not easily repaired. In relationships with less than positive or negative overarching emotional tone, one or the other person may demonstrate skills but mutual capacities are weak or absent. These dyads are at risk for sustained relationship difficulties.

This study focuses on the early experiences, inner worlds, and relational health of seventeen infants living with their incarcerated mothers in a women's correctional facility. The term "inner world" pertains to the desires, ideas, expectations, and preferences that infants conveyed through emotional expressions, shifts in attention, and a wide range of behaviors during interactions with their mothers and environment. The infants and mothers lived together in a special unit known as the Residential Parenting Program (RPP). Monday through Friday, infants also participated in an on-site Early Head Start (EHS) intervention program. Through observations and interviews that occurred over a period of 2 years, thick descriptions of infants' experiences and interactions in different contexts with their mothers and other people provided glimpses into infants' relationship experiences and inner worlds. A researcher (and the author of this report) who is a social welfare scholar, early childhood special educator, and infant mental health practitioner conducted all observations and interviews. This report focuses on two key issues: variability in early relational health for mothers and infants living in the RPP and factors that impacted infants' experiences and the development of infant–mother relationships.

Method

Qualitative methods were used to gather and analyze content from infant observations, participant observations, and interviews with infants' mothers and other caregivers. Protections for participants were reviewed and monitored by the Internal Review Board of the University of Washington.

Sources of information

Participants
Seventeen mothers and their infants participated in infant observations. Mothers were diverse in terms of race, language, ethnicity, religion, age, sexual orientation, health, social class, and culture. Ages of mothers ranged from 18 to 42 years. Ages of infants ranged from newborn to 29 months, and

41% of infants were firstborn children. At the time of this study, 34% of the infants had disabilities, Individual Family Service Plans, physical or occupational therapy, and early childhood special education services. In terms of race, 5% of infants were African American, 12% were Native American, 18% were Latino/a, 24% were mixed race, and 41% were White. Most mothers spoke English with their infants (82%). A minority (29%) had high school diplomas or GEDs at the time of their incarceration. Like most incarcerated women in the United States, these mothers struggled with addictions, posttraumatic stress, and the stress associated with life in prison (Borja et al., 2015; Fritz & Whitecare, 2016; Harris, 2014). Chemical dependency was a factor in the health of 88% of the mothers. Many mothers struggled with mental health problems: 29% had dual diagnoses, including mood disorders, and 41% had severe trauma histories and posttraumatic stress disorder.

Context

The women's correctional facility within which this study was conducted is unusual in that, despite generally operating at 117% of capacity, it offers an RPP for eligible offenders who will be released within 30 months of the birth of their infant (Condon Weisenburg, 2011; Fearn & Parker, 2004; Kopec, 2010; Quillen, 2011). A collaborative partnership between the correctional facility and a local EHS program conceived and sustains the RPP. The partnership began in 1999. The RPP allows certain pregnant offenders to return to the corrections center with their infants after delivery in a community hospital. Before acceptance into the RPP and the birth of their children, offenders must meet several criteria including (a) serving a sentence of 30 months or less; (b) completing a satisfactory essay and written application; (c) a records review that shows no outstanding warrants, no major infractions since entering the institution, no open children's protective services cases, and no convictions for violent crimes, crimes against children, or arson; (d) satisfactory in-person individual interviews with corrections counselors; and (e) an in-person interview with a panel of corrections and EHS staff.

Infants remain in their mothers' care in the RPP until their mothers' release. The RPP is segregated from the general population in the minimum security section of the corrections facility. Each mother and infant lives in an individual room. Up to 20 dyads can be enrolled in the RPP at a time. Notably, the 20 rooms that are dedicated to 20 RPP dyads are actually capable of housing 80 offenders. From the age of 6 weeks, infants are also in the care of experienced EHS infant and toddler educators in a high-quality, on-site child development center. EHS educators provide relationship-focused therapeutic care for children on Monday through Friday while their mothers are in school or at work. They also provide individual "home" visits in mothers and infants' RPP rooms, parenting classes, referrals, and other support.

The RPP aims to reduce recidivism and improve the outlook for children affected by maternal incarceration by enhancing the quality of mother–infant relationships, parenting knowledge and skills, and children's development during the first 2 years of life. Despite the many positive aspects of the RPP, prison life is stressful and particular expectations within the RPP may make it even more stressful. There are higher expectations for offenders in the RPP than there are for offenders in the general population. The risk of expulsion from the RPP constantly overshadows mothers and infants. Sometimes an offender in the RPP is demoted for rule infractions before she and her child complete the program. In this case, mother and child are immediately separated, the mother is moved to a higher-level custody unit, and the child is sent to live with someone outside the prison. Infants and mothers cannot return to the RPP after expulsion. Despite many stressors, most mothers complete the program with their children, and after release most have not returned to prison (Fearn & Parker, 2004; Kopec, 2010).

Data collection

The researcher used ethnographic and observational techniques (Atkinson & Hammersley, 1994; Emerson, Fretz, & Shaw, 2007) to generate "thick" descriptions of infants' experiences; circumstances in which infants in an RPP develop relationships with their mothers and other caregivers; and situated meanings of infants' behaviors (Sandelowski, 2000). Specifically, participant observation, interviews (Mishler, 1986) and a reflective technique called infant observation (Waddell, 2013) were used to gather redundant content about infants' experiences and the context within which they develop relationships with their mothers and other caregivers. Data were collected over a nearly 2-year period of weekly visits (year 1) and twice-a-month visits (year 2). Altogether, 1390 hours of participant observation, infant observations, and interviews generated 1300 pages of field notes and transcriptions.

Infant observation

Seventeen infants were observed with their mothers from birth or early infancy until the mothers were released from prison. Each observation lasted 45 minutes to 1 hour. Videotapes of observations were not allowed. To understand the situated meanings of infants' behaviors, the researcher also observed infants with other caregivers besides their mothers, for example EHS educators, incarcerated caregivers, and other RPP mothers. Each infant and mother were observed in six specific contexts: (a) first moments after birth in the hospital or the mother's return to the RPP with her newborn; (b) routine transitions, separations, and reunions; (c) intimate moments such as bathing, changing, feeding, being settled to sleep, or greeted when waking; (d) parent–child play; (e) socializing with other adults and infants; and (f) the morning of release from custody. The researcher wrote a detailed description of each observation on the day it was made (Waddell, 2013). Additional notes were made about (a) nuances in infant behaviors and indicators of degrees of attunement and synchrony in relationships; (b) infants' interests and needs; (c) adults' interests and needs; (d) the goodness of fit between infants' and mothers' needs and interests; (e) who the infant tried to engage; (6) who tried to engage the infant and for what purpose; (g) moments of engagement, responsiveness, shifts in attention, imitation, circles of communication, attachment strategies, and moments of delight, pleasure, flat affect, displeasure, distress, and extreme distress; (h) shifts in infants' emotions when they were in the presence of different people; (i) infants' temperaments; (j) mothers' temperaments; (k) the goodness of fit between infants' and mothers' temperaments and their temperament challenges; and (l) how mothers and infants managed transitions and coped with challenges. Sometimes observations were interrupted by prison-wide events like population count, staff shift changes, restricted movement, mail call, or summons to officers' stations. Depending on infants' and mothers' states after an interruption, the observation was either resumed or rescheduled.

Interviews

After each observation, mothers, other caregivers and/or EHS educators were asked questions about their experiences and their perceptions of the infant's behaviors during the observation. Examples of questions include (a) *I know my being here, watching your baby with you, is bound to change things for you and your baby. I wonder what parts of the experience that you and your baby had with one another today were typical, and what parts felt really different for you;* (b) *I saw you* (three- to five-word description of the mother's action at a particular moment in the interaction with her infant). *How did you know to do that?* (c) *What was going on for you when* (brief reference to the moment). *What do you think might have been going on for your baby at that moment?* (d) *What did you enjoy most?* (e) *What do you think your baby enjoyed most?* Responses to questions helped the researcher understand the significance of particular moments, events, activities, and interactions for mothers, and juxtapose and check their perspectives with hers. Most interviews lasted 45 minutes, with length depending mostly on the co-occurrence of aforementioned prison-wide events. Interviews were audiotaped and transcribed. Interviewees were invited to review their transcripts. All chose to do so, and few had edits. All the mothers asked to talk with the researcher about insights that came to them during the transcript review process.

Analyses

Empirical phenomenological techniques were used to analyze data in a multistep process: (a) studying first-order constructs and bracketing hypotheses; (b) constructing second order constructs; (c) checking for unintended effects; and (d) relating results to practice, policy and future research (Aspers, 2009).

Process
Structured methods of analysis were used to counterbalance relatively unstructured methods of data collection. The researcher began studying first-order constructs by rereading content and generating codes, infant by infant. Content was compared and categorized according to context, participants, events, and types of experiences, behaviors, themes in adult narratives, and themes in infants' accounts. The researcher studied (a) how infants and adults used gaze, movements, facial expressions, touch, voice, and proximity/distance to engage and disengage with one another, rises and falls in energy between them, and the rhythm of their actions and utterances; (b) initiations, responses, circles of communication, moments when adults and infants imitated one another, elaborated on their own actions or utterances, and added to the other's actions or utterances; (c) situated moments of cooperation, missteps, ruptures, and repairs; (d) how infants engaged and disengaged with different adults, and shifts in emotions and attention when a third person entered the interaction or the context changed. Second-order constructs focused on (a) the situated meanings of infants' and mothers' behaviors, activities, identities, roles, and relationships; (b) the focus and significance of infants' and adults' communicative attempts and behaviors; (c) indicators of their emotional and social experiences; (d) moments in which mothers showed awareness of their own and their child's inner worlds (reflective capacity); and (e) high-stress moments during which it was very difficult for mothers to be anything but self-centered, reactive, self-protective, or dismissive of their children's experiences. Patterns in infants' experiences were organized along continuums: (a) frequency of being held in a beloved's mind; (b) safety, comfort, and relaxation in mother's presence, or not; (c) present, inconsistent, or absent circles of security (Powell et al., 2013); (d) frequency of intrusive, distressing experiences with mothers and other adults, being shown off or being handed to a relative stranger, versus being protected and transferred from the arms of one familiar, safe adult to the arms of another familiar, safe adult; and (e) frequency of moments of serenity, confusion, fear, anger, or despair. The process of toggling between content grouped by codes and coded content (Sandelowski & Barroso, 2003) led to understanding of the phenomenon of living with mother in an RPP.

Unintended effects
The researcher's presence, interest, activities, and questions combined with her nonjudgmental and reflective stance had unintended effects on participants, the

research process, and context. For example, incarcerated mothers, other offenders, officers, counselors, and educators who watched the researcher watch infants and heard her wonder with adults about infants' experiences were curious. Several asked, "What is the baby saying now?" or "What do you think she's thinking or feeling?" and moved to the researcher's side as if trying to see the infant's behavior or experience from a new perspective. Many said they had never thought about babies having thoughts, ideas, or perspectives. The presence of a civilian researcher, interested in infants' and adults' perspectives, who positioned incarcerated mothers as experts and valuable informants precipitated shifts in discourses and practices (Condon Weisenburg, 2011). It also created tension. Corrections administrators and long-term (non-RPP) inmates repeatedly asked the researcher, "Why not just tell them (or us) what to do?"

Bias and trustworthiness

Given her training and experience, the researcher was predisposed to see and think about a variety of issues in ways that influenced her impressions and interpretations. These include dynamics of rank and status, marginalization and oppression; infants' welfare; developmental differences; secure, insecure, and disorganized attachment strategies; evidence of trauma, resilience, chemical dependency, and mental health and illness; and differences in executive functioning and reflective capacities among participants. Further, at the beginning of her work, the researcher was naive about prison environments and routines; corrections systems; the dynamics of life in a women's prison; competing discourses within a prison containing an RPP unit; and meanings associated with her position as a civilian researcher in a prison (Byrne, 2005; Harris, 2014; Tewksbury & Dabney, 2009). Thus, at times it was difficult for the researcher to maintain a reflective stance. Attempts were made to moderate researcher bias through (a) monthly reflective supervision; (b) using a diverse participant–stakeholder advisory board as the hub for discussion about content and process; (c) building an audit trail to cross-check data and document steps in the analytic process; (d) data triangulation; and (e) soliciting participants' help in making meaning of observations and narratives and judging the plausibility of conclusions. Reflexivity, sustained attention to relationships with participants, social context, and evidence of unintended consequences of research contribute to the trustworthiness (validity) of results (Creswell, 2003; Stige, Malterud, & Midtgarden, 2009).

Results

Overall well-being

The general context of the RPP was positive and remained that way throughout the course of the study. Infants lived, slept, and played in safe, pleasant indoor and outdoor spaces specially designed for infants, toddlers, and mothers. A dedicated pediatrician visited the infants and mothers in the RPP monthly and saw infants and mothers in a community clinic as needed between times. All received therapeutic childcare through EHS. Every mother and infant had an EHS educator who held them in mind, supported and coached mothers in understanding, caring for, and relating with their infants. EHS educators, corrections officers, and counselors monitored infants' well-being daily. Infants had active and engaging day-to-day lives and appeared to be cared for well.

Relational health

Every infant in this study remained in the RPP until at least 8 months of age and was clearly attached to at least one adult who served as a secure base and safe haven in daily life (Powell et al., 2013), meaning all infants had at least one relationship that heartened their development and internal model of attachment. Over half of the infants had consistently heartening relationships with two or more adults. Nearly 25% of infants only demonstrated secure attachment and positive relational health with an EHS educator or incarcerated caregiver who would not remain in their lives after their mothers' release from custody. In terms of infant–mother relational health, 12% of mothers and infants showed clear signs of positive relational health by 6 months of age. Over the course of time in the program, 47% of infants had mothers who became increasingly able to be emotionally present, calm, reassuring, and positively connected with them during daily routines. These mothers and infants became increasingly interested in one another's ideas, communication, and feelings. They invited responses from one another with nearly equal frequency and dominance as if they were accustomed to receiving positive responses to their attempts at engagement. These infants delighted in their mothers and felt their mothers delight in them. They tended to be calm, well-regulated infants. In contrast, 30% of infants had persistent unpredictable, less-satisfying relationships with their mothers and frequent experiences of dysregulation in their mothers' presence. In these cases, mutual interest waned and shifted to relationships with other people, and ambivalence or avoidance developed. At time of release, 18% of mothers and infants had robust positive relational health, 41% had positive relational health, and 41% remained at risk for relational health problems. The most meaningful, relevant, and differentiating aspect between infants' experiences was the extent to which their mothers were able to relate with them in authentic, healthy, and sustainable ways. Links were discovered between infants' and mothers' relational health, individual characteristics, and factors in the social environment that heartened, stalled, or thwarted infants' abilities to develop and sustain relationships.

Multiple caregivers

Attachment relationships for infants in the RPP develop in the context of multiple caregivers (Howes, 1999). The RPP is made up of a group of people who, despite having some characteristics in common, are thrown together by circumstance into close proximity and expected to function as a wholesome community. For some, but not all, participants, the RPP feels like a family. A family systems perspective is useful and relevant for considering what occurs over the course of mother–infant involvement in the program. The researcher saw shifts in relational health and dyadic functioning when the makeup of the cohort of RPP mothers and infants shifted as some were released and others were born. Thus, infants' experiences of "family" varied. Some RPP cohorts maintained a generally serene, predictable environment for infants and created a sense of community for mothers and children. Other cohorts were prone to drama, loud verbal altercations, unpredictability, and instability in adult relationships, resulting in greater irritability, neediness, and reactivity among their infants and high risk of disrupted infant–mother relationships secondary to demotions for infractions.

Reflective capacity

Mothers' responses to interview questions after infant observations revealed variations in their reflective capacities and mental states that corroborated indicators of positive and less-than-positive relational health. For example, mothers who struggled to identify and talk about their own feelings also struggled to remain sufficiently emotionally present to recognize and respond contingently to their infants' cues. Mothers who were able to respond to EHS educators' coaching and prompts to reflect on their infants' and their own experiences during play or childcare routines were more likely to enjoy interacting with their infants and sustain cycles of reciprocal responding that are essential for robust relational health. Some mothers were preoccupied or experienced diffuse distress or flashbacks to trauma during childcare routines like nursing or bottle-feeding, bathing, settling to sleep, and separations. These mothers tended to get angry with or avoid their infants, get other RPP mothers or caregivers to care for their infants, and (when their infants were calm and satisfied) ask them, "Do you love me?"

Two case studies

Contrasts in relational health are presented in Table 1. One is an example of positive-to-robust relational health; the other is an example of less than positive-to-worrisome relational health. "Penny" and "Tommy" are not the infants' real names. Both mothers were personable, single parents who had

Table 1. Variations in Relational Health.

	Penny (at 6 months)	Tommy (at 18 months)
Overarching emotion in interactions	Positive to clearly positive	Less than positive to negative
	Smiles on both faces; pleasant expressions; gentle touches; snuggling; relaxed postures; frequent eye contact; positive tones of voice and words. Penny is readily soothed. She reaches for mother and mother often leans towards her. Clear sense of safety in relationship.	Frequent flat facial expressions, frowns or grimaces on both faces. Mutual avoidance. Tommy is wary and stays out of mother's arms' reach. Mother scolds; teases; uses sarcasm and rough touch; attributes negative intents to Tommy's actions, expressions. Clear sense mother is not a secure base/safe haven.
Mutual capacities during interactions	**Always observed**: Mutual engagement, enjoyment, responsiveness, pacing, attention, initiation **Sometimes observed**: Mutual imitation	**Sometimes observed**: Mutual engagement, responsiveness, attention, initiation, shared goal, complex communication **Rarely or never observed**: Mutual enjoyment, pacing, imitation, cooperation, recognition of other's affect, coping with a challenge, shared pretend play
	Penny's mother is emotionally present, supporting, touching and responding to infant's expressions, interests, vocalizations, and movements. There are moments of fussiness with quick recovery to calm, positive emotional experience. Penny and her mother respond to each other with changes in affect, attention and energy. They often delight in one another and reach for each other. They pay more attention to each other than to objects. Penny explores; notices her mother's attention; and builds on her support and energy. Her mother often imitates her vocalizations, and Penny repeats in a back and forth volley.	There are moments of eye contact, smiles and connection but generally separateness. Tommy and his mother react to one another. She ignores; questions or demands. He responds inconsistently to his mother's commands, invitations or guidance. Circles of communication do not last long. They can play in parallel but not interactively. Tommy sometimes initiates interests, but his mother responds inconsistently. They are often out of synch, and pay more attention to objects than each other. Tommy often watches his mother from a distance. His mother is often preoccupied. There are frequent snubs. Transitions are difficult for both.
Relational health (RH) summary	Infant–mother RH: **Positive to robust** Infant–EHS educator RH: **Positive** Infant–RPP caregiver RH: **Positive** Infant–grandmother RH: **Positive**	Toddler–mother RH: **High risk** for problems Toddler–EHS educator RH: **Positive** Toddler–RPP caregiver RH: **At risk** for problems No relationships outside the RPP before release

high school diplomas or GEDs before incarceration. Both were incarcerated for nonviolent felony offenses. Both were active participants in the EHS program, earned college credits, and completed vocational training during incarceration.

Variability in relational health

An infant's mother, EHS educator. and incarcerated caregiver are the most constant people during an infant's daily life in the RPP. Other adults may be involved as well, but sporadically. For example, 41% of the infants had periodic opportunities to interact with grandparents, aunts, and siblings in a community room in the facility on visitation days and outside the facility on weekend excursions. Few had weekly or monthly visits that would enable relationships to truly develop. Some had no visitors. While she and her mother lived in the RPP, Penny had the opportunity to developing a heartening relationship with another person (her grandmother) who continued to be in her life on a daily basis after she and her mother were released. Tommy did not have a similar opportunity. By the time Penny was 11 months old, she was clearly using her mother as a secure base and safe haven (Powell et al., 2013). Penny and her mother behaved as if they felt safe, comfortable, and relaxed in each other's presence. There was clear mutual enjoyment. When Penny's mother came to pick her up from care, she smiled and approached Penny with open arms. Penny smiled in return or showed off, then crawled directly to her mother's arms. Adults smiled and commented on how happy Penny was to see her mommy. Penny's and her mother's interest in and affection for one another continued for the duration of their time in the RPP. At 11 months of age, Tommy could crawl faster than he could walk. When he saw his mother enter a room to pick him up, he immediately dropped to his knees; crawled quickly and silently to a far point in the room, and then turned, sat, and solemnly watched his mother from a distance for 3 minutes or longer. His mother greeted adults and sought their attention instead of his attention. Adults' attention invariably shifted from Tommy to his mother. Tommy's mother often snubbed him by glancing toward him then warmly greeting other children and offering them toys, hugs, and attention. On the rare occasions that she approached him, Tommy determinedly evaded his mother, crawled to the arms or legs of another caregiver, or got busy playing elsewhere. Time and again, adults either did not notice Tommy's behavior or interpreted Tommy's avoidance as independence, "flirting," reluctance to leave "school," or being a "typical" active boy. Adults seemed unable to see the reunification ritual from Tommy's perspective or its significance for his future well-being. Both dyads were considered successes at the time of their release from custody for the following reasons. Both mothers completed college and training during their time in the program, meaning they had good employment prospects after release. Both had infraction-free records. Both left with healthy, typically developing, personable children. Six years after release, Penny, her mother, and their relationship are thriving. They are well connected to a network of positive formal and informal supports. Within a month of release, Tommy had begun experiencing a series of traumatic events and periods of abandonment and neglect. Less than 1 year after release, Tommy's mother was reincarcerated and he entered the child welfare system. Predictors of incarcerated parents' "success" after release do not necessarily align with predictors of infants' well-being.

Discussion

The purpose of this study was to document infants' early experiences and situated behaviors while living with their incarcerated mothers in an RPP, to understand their inner worlds and relational health. Despite a general context that remained positive throughout the course of the study, results showed variability in infants' experiences and relational health. Infant, mother, and larger systemic contributions to variability will be discussed categorically.

Infants' contributions

Infants' contributions to variability in their experiences and relational health were constitutional and maturational, namely the influence of health status at a given time on their energy, sense of ease in their bodies, and ability to breathe comfortably, sleep, eat, eliminate, move, and experience increasingly longer periods of calm alertness, pleasure, and regulation. These factors and temperament influenced infants' capacity for engagement, attention, enjoyment, and responsiveness to their mothers, other caregivers, and environment. The infants in this study were generally healthy. With one exception, none required special handling or sensitivity. Fortunately, in that case, the mother felt a strong bond with her infant, was emotionally present, enjoyed her infant, was exceptionally responsive to EHS educators' coaching, and steadily grew adept and confident in mothering her infant.

Mothers' contributions

Mothers' contributions to variability in infants' experiences and relational health are organized into five categories, namely the RPP mother's (a) health, (b) mindfulness, (c) relationship with her infant, (d) relationships with others, and (e) anticipation of a supporting matrix after release. Definitive examples of themes are presented in Table 2.

Table 2. Maternal Factors that Contributed to Infant–Mother Relational Health in the RPP.

Mother's health
Mother's physical and mental health and general well-being
The presence or absence of postnatal depression
Ongoing access to mental health care including timely prescription refills during incarceration
Sturdiness of recovery from chemical dependency, and awareness of triggers for relapse
Progress in transcending past traumas

Mother's mindfulness
Capacity for honesty, self-awareness, self-compassion, perspective taking, and impulse control
Ability to tune into her own needs, experiences in her body, emotions and thought patterns
Ability to self-regulate and help her infant be regulated during moments of stress
How mother reorganizes her identity during her time in the RPP

Mother's relationship with her infant
How predictably, accurately and sensitively mother interprets and responds her infant's cues
Ability to be emotionally present and to comfort her crying, fussy or irritable infant
Ability to think about her infant's temperament, experiences, feelings, and perspective
Continuity of access to a person with a positive internal model of infant–mother relationships who can support interactions when mother and infant struggle to relate with one another
Ways in which mother moves through space and social circles in the prison with her infant
How mother transfers her infant into the arms of another person and whether the other person is someone with whom her infant has a wholesome relationship
Extent to which mother intentionally protects her infant from exposure to interactions between offenders, or offenders and officers, that might be confusing or distressing for an infant

Mother's relationships with others
How mother relates to adults when her infant is and is not present, and to her infant when other adults and children are and are not present
Ability to respond to, relate and cooperate with other RPP mothers, other offenders, officers, counselors, and educators (as opposed to reacting, opposing, bargaining, or avoiding)
Motivation and ability to safeguard her relationship with her infant by not acting out, intentionally breaking rules or otherwise jeopardizing their time and place in the RPP
Reactions to shifts in status, rank, social dynamics, and rules in the RPP
Reactions when other mothers and infants come and go from the RPP

Mother's anticipation of a supporting matrix post-release
Anticipation of safety, security, and community support after release
Opportunities and ability to start building healthy relationships with people who will support the tough internal work and lifestyle changes that will be necessary to sustain sobriety, mental health, balance, and infant–mother relational health after release

Mothers' mental health affects infants' mental health and relational health. Sadly, the mental health system in the facility was overburdened during the time of this study, in part due to crowding in the prison. Priority access to mental health clinicians was understandably directed toward severe, acute cases that adversely affect custody unit functioning and offenders' and officers' safety. Consequently, when the system was particularly overburdened, there were lapses of 2 weeks or longer between refills for offenders' prescriptions. When RPP mothers with mood disorders experienced lapses in medication regimens, they were at risk for demotion and expulsion from the RPP, secondary to severe emotional dysregulation, ups and downs in mania, and depression. Their infants were confused and distressed. During these periods, infants' well-being depended on others' willingness and ability to calm them and care for them. It took time and effort to repair ruptures that happened in these infant–mother relationships. Some were able to repair ruptures in 5 or 6 weeks, which is nonetheless a significant length of time in an infant's life. Others needed more time and extra support from EHS educators. Infants' life experiences are inextricably tied to their relationship experiences (Bowlby, 1988; Stern, 1985), meaning infants understand adults' behavior as a reflection of themselves. In the early months of life, infants do not differentiate adults' actions from how those actions make them feel. Over time, their experiences during interactions with their parents become a blueprint or inner working model for their developing sense of self, and set the stage for later relationship patterns (Cicchetti et al., 2006; Fraiberg et al., 1975; Lieberman & Amaya-Jackson, 2005; Osofsky, 2004). Consistent access to mental health care for parents and infants is needed when intermittent mental illness, chemical dependency relapse, hidden traumas or intergenerational patterns of difficulties in early relationships are a concern. This was the case for nearly nine of every ten infant-mother dyads in this study. A heartening factor in RPP infants' experiences may be their mothers' reasons for hope for their futures and their ability to envision better relationships with their children than they had with their parents. Mothers in this study who anticipated safety, security, and community support for lifestyle changes they began during their time in the RPP had more positive outlooks in general; they were more likely to be self-compassionate; to talk about fears, plans and resources; to enjoy their infants; and to help their infants form healthy attachments with people who would remain in their lives after release.

Caregivers' contributions

EHS educators and some incarcerated caregivers were able to serve as secure bases and safe havens for infants (Powell et al., 2013). This was an important relational health safety net for all the infants, particularly when infants and mothers struggled to relate with one another. For at least 8 months, every infant in this study had recurring opportunities to develop a positive sense of self, trust, emotional capacities, and skills they could use to generalize a positive model for relationships to future relationships. Some people question the merit of allowing infants to live with incarcerated mothers (Unity, 2001). In this study, every infant had positive to robust relational health with at least one adult. Neurodevelopmentally speaking, positive early parent- or caregiver–child relationships directly affect brain development and serve as a protective factor in future development and relationships.

System-level contributions

System-level contributions to infants' early experiences and relational health included (a) the corrections system's commitment to sustaining a high-quality RPP; (b) the presence of on-site therapeutic care for infants in a high-quality EHS child development center; (c) ongoing collaboration between EHS and corrections personnel even when systems were under stress; (d) collaboration between corrections counselors, EHS educators and a community-based statewide organization of volunteers who helped many (but not all) of the mothers prepare for release in practical ways and generally made a commitment to remain connected with infants and mothers during their transition back to their local communities; and (e) corrections and EHS system's willingness to collaborate in an intense, qualitative, participatory study of the experiences and relational health of infants in their care. As findings emerged, corrections officers and other stakeholders imagined, advocated for, and enacted systems change, for example, revising internal RPP protocols and procedures and launching a statewide alternative sentencing program for mothers and fathers (Aguiar & Leavell, 2017).

Limitations

This study has several limitations. Data included thick descriptions of infant–mother interactions that included indications of relational health, but the researcher did not specifically collect relational health assessment data through standardized means. This study did not include following infants, mothers, and their relationships after release. Despite a desire to do so, the researcher was not able to videotape infant–mother interactions, watch them with mothers, and collect data about mother's reflections while watching their interactions. The researcher did not gather data across mothers about their inner working models of attachment, reflective capacities, physical, mental and relational health histories, and current status. Collectively, these additional data would provide some insight into the relationship models infants might develop. The incarcerated mothers of infants in this study feared and talked about the ever-present danger of making mistakes, receiving infractions, having to leave the RPP, and losing their children. These and other anxieties affected their mental states, ruminations, daydreams and nightmares, conversations, responses during interviews, and behavior. Prudence is needed in generalizing findings to other settings and populations.

Conclusion

This study adds consideration of relational health constructs to the literature on children of incarcerated parents. Variability in infants' experiences and relational health in an RPP has implications for social work practice, policy, and research. Systems could maximize relational health benefits to infants and toddlers who live with incarcerated parents by implementing collaborative cross-agency programs with aims that include positive early relational health, participation in EHS or other infant–parent programs, and making prerelease planning for continued stability and positive relational health after release a priority. Crafting a supportive postrelease matrix for RPP infants and mothers means (a) making sure that there will be a smooth, immediate transfer to a EHS program, pediatrician, and a mental health care provider and (b) identifying a family member, friend, or community volunteer who demonstrates capacity for positive relational health with the infant before release and makes a commitment to remaining in the infant's life post-release. For different reasons, despite the quality of the programs, indicators of relational health for infants in this study were not apparent to the pediatrician, RPP counselors, and EHS educators who worked with them. If routine relational health assessments were a part of EHS services, parents, EHS educators, and RPP counselors would have opportunities to see strengths, vulnerabilities and change over time, and use the information to help them work with community providers in planning for release. Early indicators of relational health can be readily observed *in vivo* and in brief video clips by nonresearchers. Practitioners can learn to watch and discuss observations with parents and use parents' reflections to guide strengths-based, relational health-focused interventions (Condon et al., 2016). Weekly or biweekly consultation with an infant and early childhood mental health consultant would be a protective measure for children because (a) consultation would support counselors, officers, educators, parents, and other stakeholders in thinking about different levels of influence in difficult situations, interpersonal dynamics, and children's well-being; (b) help parents make choices that promote and protect their children's physical, mental, and relational health; (c) help stakeholders implement child- and relational health-centered decision-making; and (d) give stakeholders an indicator of the success of their efforts to promote stability for children and families affected by parental incarceration. Johnston and Brinamen (2006) describe a consultation model that could be adapted for use in prison- and community-based settings that aim to promote relational health and enduring benefits for infants, young children, and parents.

Jones Harden (2007) described infants' experiences in the child welfare system and suggested action steps to enhance their well-being. Her work mobilized and helped focus the efforts of advocates to change an overburdened and struggling system of care. This study is a step toward a similar treatise on behalf of infants whose lives are linked with corrections systems. Better understanding is needed of (a) the early experiences and relational health of infants and toddlers who remain in the care of their incarcerated parents; (b) associations between discourses in settings where infants and incarcerated parents receive services, parents' states of mind, and infants' and parents' relational health; (c) parallel processes of change and relational health outcomes in programs that do and do not embed infant and early childhood mental health consultation and reflective practices in their operations; and (d) longitudinal studies of the relational health of infants of incarcerated parents. The capacity of infants' accounts to facilitate change in practices, policies, and systems will depend on the usefulness and relevance of findings of future phenomenological and mixed-methods studies to various communities of practice, particularly for the most vulnerable and marginalized populations of infants and parents.

References

Aguiar, C. M., & Leavell, S. (2017). A statewide parenting alternative sentencing program: Description and initial outcomes. *Smith College Studies in Social Work, 87*(1), 78–94.

Ainsworth, M. D., Blehar, M. C., Waters, E., & Wall, S. (1978). *Patterns of attachment: A psychological study of the strange situation*. Hillside, NJ: Lawrence Erlbaum Associates.

Aspers, P. (2009). Empirical phenomenology: A qualitative research approach. *Indo-Pacific Journal of Phenomenology, 9*(2), 1–12. doi:10.1080/20797222.2009.11433992

Atkinson, P., & Hammersley, M. (1994). Ethnography and participant observation. In N. K. Densin, & Y. S. Lincoln (Eds.), *Handbook of qualitative research* (pp. 248–261). Thousand Oaks, CA: Sage Publications.

Baradon, T., Fonagy, P., Bland, K., Lenard, K., & Sleed, M. (2008). New beginnings: An experience-based programme addressing the attachment relationship between mothers and their babies in prisons. *Journal of Child Psychotherapy, 34*(2), 240–258. doi:10.1080/00754170802208065

Belsky, J. (1999). Interactional and contextual determinants of attachment security. In J. C. Cassidy, & P. R. Shaver (Eds.), *Handbook of attachment: Theory, research, and clinical applications* (pp. 249–264). New York, NY: Guilford Press.

Berlin, L. J., Ziv, L., Amaya-Jackson, M., & Greenberg, M. T. (Eds.). (2005). *Enhancing early attachments: Theory, research, intervention, and policy*. New York, NY: The New Press.

Berry, P., & Eigenberg, H. (2003). Role strain and incarcerated mothers: Understanding the process of mothering. *Women & Criminal Justice, 15*(1), 101–119. doi:10.1300/J012v15n01_06

Bick, E. (1987). Notes on infant observation in psychoanalytic training. In M. H. Williams (Ed.), *Collected papers of Martha Harris and Esther Bick* (pp. 240–256). London, UK: Clunie Press. (Original work published 1964)

Borelli, J. L., Goshin, L., Joestl, S., Clark, J., & Byrne, M. W. (2010). Attachment organization in a sample of incarcerated mothers: Distribution of classifications and associations with substance abuse history, depressive symptoms, perceptions of parenting competency and social support. *Attachment & Human Development, 12*(4), 355–374. doi:10.1080/14616730903416971

Borja, S., Nurius, P., & Eddy, J. M. (2015). Adversity across the life course of incarcerated parents: Gender differences. *Journal of Forensic Social Work, 5*(1–3), 167–185. doi:10.1080/1936928X.2015.1093992

Bowlby, J. (1988). *A secure base: Parent-child attachment and healthy human development.* New York, NY: Basic Books.

Brazelton, T. B., & Cramer, B. G. (1990). *The earliest relationship: Parents, infants and the drama of early attachment.* Reading, MA: Perseus Books.

Byrne, M. W. (2005). Conducting research as a visiting scientist in a women's prison. *Journal of Professional Nursing, 21*(4), 223–230. doi:10.1016/j.profnurs.2005.05.001

Byrne, M. W., Goshin, L. S., & Joestl, S. (2010). Intergenerational transmission of attachment for infants raised in a prison nursery. *Attachment & Human Development, 12*(4), 375–393. doi:10.1080/14616730903417011

Cassidy, J. (1999). The nature of the child's ties. In J. Cassidy, & P. R. Shaver (Eds.), *Handbook of attachment: Theory, research, and clinical applications,* (pp. 3–20). New York, NY: Guilford Press.

Cassidy, J., Poehlmann, J., & Shaver, P. R. (2010). An attachment perspective on incarcerated parents and their children. *Attachment & Human Development, 12*(4), 285–288. doi:10.1080/14616730903417110

Cassidy, J., Ziv, Y., Stupica, B., Sherman, L. J., Butler, H., Karfgin, A. ... Powell, B. (2010). Enhancing maternal sensitivity and attachment security in the infants of women in a jail-diversion program. *Attachment I Human Development, 12*(4), 333–353.

Cicchetti, D., Rogosch, F. A., & Toth, S. L. (2006). Fostering secure attachment in infants in maltreating families through preventive interventions. *Development and Psychopathology, 18,* 623–649. doi:10.1017/S0954579406060329

Condon, M.-C., Carver, M., Crawley, P., Freeman, E., & Van Cleave, S. (2010, November). *Research and action in Washington's prison nursery.* Presented at The Portia Project Criminal Justice Conference, Eugene, OR.

Condon, M.-C., Willis, D. W., & Eddy, J. M. (2016). *Early relational health assessment and reflective practice.* Unpublished manuscript.

Condon Weisenburg, M.-C. (2011). *Speaking of babies: Participatory action research in a prison nursery.* Bellingham, WA: Applied Digital Imaging.

Creswell, J. W. (2003). *Research design: Qualitative, quantitative, and mixed methods approaches* (2nd ed.). Thousand Oaks, CA: Sage Publications.

Crittenden, P. M. (2008). *Raising parents: Attachment, parenting and child safety.* New York, NY: Willan Publishing.

Crittenden, P. M., & Claussen, A. H. (Eds.). (2000). *The organization of attachment relationships: Maturation, culture, and context.* New York, NY: Cambridge University Press.

Crittenden, P. M., & Landini, A. (2011). *Assessing adult attachment: A dynamic-maturational approach to discourse analysis.* New York, NY: W.W. Norton & Company.

Eddy, J. M., Martinez, C. R., Schiffmann, T., Newton, R., Olin, L., Leve, L. ... Shortt, J. W. (2008). Development of a multisystemic parent management training intervention for incarcerated parents, their children and families. *Clinical Psychologist, 12*(3), 86–98. doi:10.1080/13284200802495461

Emerson, R., Fretz, R. I., & Shaw, L. (2007). *Writing ethnographic fieldnotes.* Chicago, IL: University of Chicago Press.

Fearn, N. E., & Parker, K. (2004). Washington State's residential parenting program: An integrated public health, education, and social service resource for pregnant inmates and prison mothers. *Californian Journal of Health Promotion, 2*(4), 34–48.

Fraiberg, S., Adelson, E., & Shapiro, V. (1975). Ghosts in the nursery: A psychoanalytic approach to the problems of impaired infant-mother relationships. *Child & Adolescent Psychiatry, 14*(3), 387–421.

Fritz, S., & Whitecare, K. (2016). Prison nurseries: Experiences of incarcerated women during pregnancy. *Journal of Offender Rehabilitation, 55*(1), 1–20. doi:10.1080/10509674.2015.1107001

Goshin, L. S., & Byrne, M. W. (2009). Converging streams of opportunity for prison nursery programs in the United States. *Journal of Offender Rehabilitation, 48*, 271–295. doi:10.1080/10509670902848972

Harris, M. S. (2014). Group therapy at a prison for women: A therapist's perspective. *Smith College Studies in Social Work, 84*(1), 40–54. doi:10.1080/00377317.2014.862114

Howes, C. (1999). Attachment relationships in the context of multiple caregivers. In J. C. Cassidy, & P. R. Shaver (Eds.), *Handbook of attachment: Theory, research and clinical applications* (pp. 671–687). New York, NY: Guilford Press.

Johnson, S. C., Dweck, C. S., & Chen, F. S. (2007). Evidence for infants' internal working models of attachment. *Psychology Science, 18*(6), 501–502. doi:10.1111/j.1467-9280.2007.01929.x

Johnston, K., & Brinamen, C. (2006). *Mental health consultation in childcare: Transforming relationships among directors, staff, and families.* Washington, DC: Zero to Three.

Jones Harden, B. (2007). *Infants in the child welfare system: A developmental framework for policy and practice.* Washington, DC: Zero to Three.

Karen, R. (1994). *Becoming attached: First relationships and how they shape our capacity to love.* New York, NY: Oxford University Press.

Katz, L. F., Lederman, C. S., & Osofsky, J. D. (2011). *Child-centered practices for the courtroom and community: A guide to working effectively with young children and their families in the child welfare system.* Baltimore, MD: Paul H. Brookes Publishing Company, Inc.

Kjellstrand, J. M., & Eddy, J. M. (2011). Parental incarceration during childhood, family context, and youth problem behavior across adolescence. *Journal of Offender Rehabilitation, 50*(1), 18–36. doi:10.1080/10509674.2011.536720

Kopec, D. (2010). *Purdy.* Tacoma, WA: KBTC Public Television. Retrieved from http://www.kbtc.org

Lange, S. M. (2008). The challenges confronting children of incarcerated parents. *Journal of Family Psychotherapy, 11*(4), 61–68. doi:10.1300/J085v11n04_03

Lieberman, A. F. (1993). *The emotional life of the toddler.* New York, NY: The Free Press.

Lieberman, A. F., & Amaya-Jackson, L. (2005). Reciprocal influences of attachment and trauma: Using a dual lens in the assessment and treatment of infants, toddlers, and preschoolers. In L. J. Berlin, Y. Ziv, L. M. Amaya-Jackson, & M. T. Greenberg (Eds.), *Enhancing early attachments: Theory research, intervention and policy* (pp. 100–125). New York, NY: Guilford Press.

Lombardi, J., & Bogle, M. M. (Eds.). (2004). *Beacon of hope.* Washington, DC: Zero to Three.

Makariev, D. W., & Shaver, P. R. (2010). Attachment, parental incarceration and possibilities for intervention: An overview. *Attachment & Human Development, 12*(4), 311–331. doi:10.1080/14751790903416939

McHale, J. P. (2007). When infants grow up in multiperson relationship systems. *Infant Mental Health Journal, 28*(4), 370–392. doi:10.1002/(ISSN)1097-0355

Mishler, E. G. (1986). *Research interviewing: Context and narrative.* Cambridge, MA: Harvard University Press.

Myerson, J., Otteson, C., & Ryba, K. L. (2010). *Childhood disrupted: Understanding the features and effects of maternal incarceration.* St. Paul, MN: Wilder Research.

Osofsky, J. D. (Ed.). (2004). *Young children and trauma: Intervention and treatment.* New York, NY: Guilford Press.

Pattillo, M., Weiman, D., & Western, B. (Eds.). (2004). *Imprisoning America: The social effects of mass incarceration.* New York, NY: Russell Sage Foundation.

Powell, B., Cooper, G., Hoffman, K., & Marvin, B. (2007). The circle of security project: A case study—"It hurts to give what which you did not receive." In D. Oppenheim & D. F. Goldsmith (Eds.), *Attachment theory in clinical work with children: Bridging the gap between research and practice* (pp. 172–202). New York, NY: Guilford Press.

Powell, B., Cooper, G., Hoffman, K., & Marvin, B. (2013). *The circle of security intervention: Enhancing attachment in early parent-child relationships.* New York, NY: Guilford Press.

Quillen, A. (2011, January). Raising babies in prison: Supporting the bond between inmates and their newborns gives these families a new start. *Yes! Magazine.* Retrieved from http://www.yesmagazine.org/issues/what-happy-families-know/raising-babies-in-prison

Rebecca Project for Human Rights & The National Women's Law Center. (2010). *Mothers behind bars: A state-by-state report card and analysis of federal policies on conditions of confinement for pregnant and parenting women and the effect on their children.* Washington, DC: National Women's Law Center.

Sameroff, A. J., McDonough, S. C., & Rosenblum, K. L. (Eds.). (2004). *Treating parent-infant relationship problems: Strategies for intervention.* New York, NY: Guilford Press.

Sandelowski, M. (2000). Whatever happened to qualitative description? *Research in Nursing & Health, 23,* 334–340. doi:10.1002/1098-240X(200008)23:4<334::AID-NUR9>3.0.CO;2-G

Sandelowski, M., & Borroso, J. (2003). Classifying the findings in qualitative studies. *Qualitative Health Research, 13*(7), 905–923. doi:10.1177/1049732303253488

Shlafer, R. J., & Poehlmann, J. (2010). Attachment and caregiving relationships in families affected by parental incarceration. *Attachment & Human Development, 12*(4), 395–415.

Shlafer, R. J., Raby, K. L., Laler, J. M., Hesemeyer, P. S., & Roisman, G. I. (2015). Longitudinal associations between adult attachment states of mind and parenting quality. *Attachment & Human Development, 17*(1), 83–95. doi:10.1080/14616734.2014.962064

Sleed, M., Baradon, T., & Fonagy, P. (2013). New beginnings for mothers and babies in prison: A cluster randomized control trial. *Attachment & Human Development, 15*(4), 349–367. doi:10.1080/14616734.2013.782651

Spieker, S., Nelson, E., & Condon, M.-C. (2011). Validity of the TAS-45 as a measure of toddler-parent attachment: Preliminary evidence from early Head Start families. *Attachment & Human Development, 13*(1), 69–90. doi:10.1080/14616734.2010.488124

Stern, D. N. (1985). *The interpersonal world of the infant: A view from psychoanalysis and developmental psychology.* New York, NY: Basic Books.

Stern, D. N. (1990). *Diary of a baby: What your child sees, feels, and experiences.* New York, NY: Basic Books.

Stern, D. N. (1995). *The motherhood constellation: A unified view of parent-infant psychotherapy.* New York, NY: Basic Books.

Stern, D. N. (2002). *The first relationship: Infant and mother.* Cambridge, MA: Harvard University Press.

Stige, B., Malterud, K., & Midtgarden, T. (2009). Toward an agenda for evaluation of qualitative research. *Qualitative Health Research, 19*(10), 1504–1516. doi:10.1177/1049732309348501

Tewksbury, R., & Dabney, D. (Eds.). (2009). *Prisons and jails: A reader.* New York, NY: McGraw-Hill.

Unity, A. (2001). Babies behind bars: Do babies benefit from being in prison with their mothers? *Journal of Community Care, 29,* 24–26.

Villanueva, C. (2009). *Mothers, infants and imprisonment: A national look at prison nurseries and community-based alternatives.* New York, NY: Women's Prison Association.

Waddell, M. (2013). Infant observation in Britain: A Tavistock approach. *International Journal of Infant Observation and Its Applications, 16*(1), 4–22. doi:10.1080/13698036.2013.765659

Whaley, R. B., Moe, A. M., Eddy, J. M., & Dougherty, J. (2008). The domestic violence experiences of women in community corrections. *Women & Criminal Justice, 18*(3), 25–45. doi:10.1300/J012v18n03_02

Zeanah, C. H. (2009). *Handbook of infant mental health* (3rd ed.). New York, NY: Guilford Press.

Incarcerated Mothers: Trauma and Attachment Issues

Marian S. Harris, PhD, LICSW, ACSW

ABSTRACT

Although men comprise the largest portion of the prison population in the United States, the number of women in prison has increased more than 800% during the past three decades. More than 60% of these women are mothers of children under 18 years of age. There continues to be a gap in our knowledge base regarding mothers who are incarcerated. In this study, unresolved issues of trauma and attachment are explored for 28 incarcerated mothers involved with the child welfare system. Data were collected using the Trauma Attachment and Belief Scale (TABS) and the Adult Attachment Interview (AAI). Findings from the TABS revealed scores of average and high average in beliefs related to five need areas that are sensitive to the effects of traumatic experiences, namely self-safety, self-trust, self-esteem, self-intimacy, and self-control. Most participants were classified as disorganized/disoriented based on their narrative responses to questions from the AAI protocol. Implications for the results are discussed.

The number of incarcerated mothers continues to increase in the U.S. criminal justice system, an issue of great importance to their children and families (Glaze & Maruschak, 2011; Sykes & Pettit, 2014; The Sentencing Project, 2015). According to Bowlby (1969), the mother–child attachment relationship begins in infancy and is significant across the lifespan. Children need their mothers and mothers need their children. There is no replacement for a mother. While mothers and fathers are important to children, a mother is usually the primary caregiver, especially during the early years of life.

Parental responsibilities for rearing children, which often fall to the mother, include the provision of nurturance and physical care; training and channeling of psychological needs in toilet training, weaning, solid foods, etc.; teaching and skill-training in language, perceptual skills, physical skills, self-care skills to facilitate care, ensure safety, and other important goals; orienting the child to his immediate world of kin, neighborhood, community, and society, and to his own feelings; transmitting cultural and subcultural goals and values and motivating the child to accept them for his own;

promoting interpersonal skills, motive, and modes of feeling and behaving in relation to others; and guiding, correcting, helping the child to formulate his own goals and plan his own activities (LeFlore & Holson, 1989). When a mother is incarcerated, someone else becomes the child's caregiver and takes on the aforementioned parental responsibilities.

What happens to a child varies greatly. Children may end up in the child welfare system, especially African American and Native American children (Child Welfare League of North America, 2001; Harris, 2014). Grandmothers or other close family members may assume the role of primary caregiver when a mother is incarcerated. Regardless, "the development of the representational world into a cohesive and integrated sense of reality occurs within the context of the primary caregiving relationship. Eventually this context expands to include significant others" (Blatt & Lerner, 1983, p. 25). When this relationship is disrupted, a child is in a vulnerable position. Children thrive in their growth and development when they have a loving and nurturing mother who is emotionally and physically present in their lives.

Winnicott (1956) explored the self-formation of the infant within the matrix of the mother–infant relationship. One does not have to be a perfect mother, but just—in Winnicott's famous phrase—a "good enough" mother. The mother–child relationship is disrupted whenever a mother is sent to jail or prison. This disruption affects children as well as their mothers in very deleterious ways. Mothers are faced with trauma and attachment issues including separation and loss. This paper explores the connection between unresolved loss and trauma in mothers and the resulting issues in terms of the mother–child relationship when mothers are incarcerated and involved with the child welfare system.

Background

The continued increase in the number of women in U.S. prisons and in prisons around the world is a major concern for professionals in varied disciplines including criminal justice, social work, psychology, mental health, education, child welfare, and juvenile justice. This trend has been well documented over the years (Campbell & Robinson, 1997; Carlen, 1998; Gursansky, Harvey, McGrath, & O'Brien, 1998; McGalliard, 2012; Philips & Gleeson, 2007; The Sentencing Project, 2015). The high number of incarcerated parents in this country means that a large percentage of children, especially children of color and poor children, experience the loss of their mothers and/or fathers (Sykes & Pettit, 2014). The growth rate for the imprisonment of women has outpaced that of men by more than 50% in the past three decades (The Sentencing Project, 2015, p. 1). According to Glaze and Maruschak (2011), there are more than 120,000 incarcerated mothers in the United States and 64% to 84% of mothers had at least one minor child in their care and custody before their incarceration.

Reasons for incarceration

Approximately 75% of incarcerated women are mothers. There are several common reasons why women are incarcerated. Women in state prison who are mothers are more often convicted of drug offenses (63%), property offenses (65%), and public-order offenses (65%). The 57% of women convicted of violent offenses tend not to be mothers. Further, in federal prison, a higher percentage of fathers (69%) as opposed to mothers (55%), are drug offenders (Glaze & Maruschak, 2009).

During the past few decades, the percentage of women in state prisons incarcerated for a drug offense has doubled (The Sentencing Project, 2015). This increase is the result of the "war on drugs" and the tough on crime policies that currently prevail in this country. President Nixon declared this war in the early 1970s. Initial efforts included a large increase in federal drug control agencies as well as mandatory sentencing and no-knock warrants. These efforts were expanded during the presidency of Ronald Reagan. One result was that the number of people incarcerated for nonviolent drug law offenses increased from 50,000 in 1980 to more than 400,000 by 1997. Subsequently, "zero tolerance" policies were implemented in the mid-to-late 1980s. The prison population continued to increase because of public and political hysteria regarding drugs, which led to the passage of a set of draconian anti-drug acts. These acts greatly affected the lives of the many mothers who are incarcerated for drug offenses.

> Other efforts to explain the sharp increase in women's imprisonment have focused on the 'war on drugs,' with its emphasis on street-level sweeps of those engaged in the drug trade and harsh mandatory sentencing. The crackdown on drug crime was sold to the American public as the answer to an escalating epidemic of male violence. Yet despite their roles as relatively minor players in the drug trade, women-disproportionate numbers of them, African American and Latina, have been 'caught in the net' of increasingly punitive policing, prosecutorial, and sentencing policies (Harrison & Beck, 2007). Once in the system, women often have little choice but to accept plea bargains and then face mandatory minimum sentencing laws that restrict judges from mitigating the impact of their sentencing decisions in consideration of their family situations or their obvious need for substance abuse treatment (Frost, Greene, & Pranis, 2006, pp. 23–24).

Incarcerated mothers and fathers pay a high price for drug offenses; this price is also seen in the ways their lives are affected by varied policies after they are released from prison. For example, the "one strike" law regarding drug use allows public housing authorities throughout the United States to deny admission or terminate assistance to illegal drug users and alcohol abusers; this includes guests in a household. The Housing Opportunity Act of 1996 and the Quality Housing and Work Responsibility Act of 1998 give much latitude to local housing authorities in determining eligibility for Section 8 and several other federally assisted housing programs; these local authorities determine the type of crimes that will make an applicant ineligible for public housing programs and the length of time to deny people with criminal records housing assistance (Mukamal & Samuels, 2002). The extent and ramification of these policies adversely impact the lives of incarcerated mothers once they are released from state or federal prisons.

Trauma and attachment issues

Trauma, in its varied forms, has been shown to form the foundation for a new paradigm for understanding and addressing psychopathology and the ability for safe and effective parenting. An integration of the advances of neuroscience and the study of early attachment relationships form the foundation for this paradigm (Schore, 1994, 2003). Trauma can profoundly affect one's life trajectory. According to Freud (1917, 1963), psychic trauma occurs when an individual experiences an acute, overwhelming threat. The trauma affects the individual's psychological base, which is grounded in a secure sense of past occurrences and a current state of being (Erikson, 1968). "Trauma" refers to any event that threatens the life of an individual or a loved one. One can experience chronic trauma and/or complex trauma. Chronic trauma is a recurring event that occurs over a prolonged period of time. However, complex trauma occurs as a result of a chronic traumatic event and the emotional as well as physical impact.

In thinking about mothers who are incarcerated, this paradigm would begin by asking the question: What traumas or losses have they experienced in their lives? Examples might include the following: the death of a parent, abandonment by a parent, severe neglect, and sexual or physical abuse by a parent or stranger. The effect of early abuse and neglect is the formation of a disorganized-disoriented attachment, which is evident during the latter stages of childhood, adolescence, and adulthood, and serves as a risk factor for future psychiatric disorders (Schore, 2001; Carrion et al., 2001). Early maltreatment in childhood, especially sexual abuse and psychological neglect/parental disattunement, negatively affects early parent–child attachment and can cause problems in interpersonal relationships (Caffey, 1965; 1972). The formation of internal working models of attachment is affected by the quality of early parenting and influences a child's later relational behavior with her/his mother as well as with others. There is an intergenerational concordance in relationship patterns, which has been documented in epidemiological research studies (Frommer & O'Shea, 1973; Rutter & Liddle, 1983; Rutter & Madge, 1976). Fraiberg, Adelson, and Shapiro (1975) demonstrated how a parent's past can influence the parent–child relationship during the child's early developmental stages.

> In every nursery there are ghosts. There are the visitors from the unremembered past of the parents; the uninvited guests at the christening.... Even among families where the loved ones are stable and strong the intruders from the parental past may break through the magic circle in an unguarded moment, and a parent and his child may find themselves reenacting a moment or scene from another time with another set of characters.... Another group of families appear to be possessed by their ghosts. The intruders from the past have taken up residence in their nursery claiming tradition and rights of ownership. They have been present at the christening for two or more generations. While none has issued an invitation the ghosts take up residence and conduct the rehearsal of the family tragedy from a tattered script (pp. 387–388).

Mothers who have been neglected, abused, and deprived seem to experience problems in parent–child attachment, especially when they do not have an opportunity to resolve the problems/issues that result from these traumatic experiences; consequently, an intergenerational cycle of unresolved trauma is set into motion. A frequent outcome of child maltreatment in high-risk adults is unresolved trauma (Berthelot et al., 2015; Iyengar, Kim, Martinez, Fonagy, & Stratheam, 2014; Murphy et al., 2014; Riggs et al., 2007; Stovall-McClough & Cloitre, 2006). It is important to understand the intergenerational transmission of attachment in abused and neglected mothers (Harris, 2011).

Attachment theory focuses on one's early relationships. The premise of Bowlby's (1969, 1988) theory of attachment is that one's attachment to a primary caregiver during the first year of life has significant outcomes throughout the life span. If the attachment relationship is secure and positive the individual will have optimal development; however, if the attachment relationship is insecure and negative the individual's development is not likely to be optimal (Bowlby, 1969, 1989). There are two frames that are essential to understanding attachment across the life span. First, it is highly significant to understand internal working models of attachment and individual differences in security and anxiety; second, it is essential to understand that a child's sense of security and safety is based on the availability and responsiveness of attachment figures (Bowlby, 1973).

Findings from previous research have revealed that patterns of sensitive responsiveness results in intergenerational secure attachment based on studies using the Adult Attachment Interview (AAI) (Ainsworth, Blehar, Waters, & Wall, 1978; George, 1984; George, Kaplan, & Main, 1984; George & Solomon, 1996). There has also been research regarding patterns of intergenerational insecure attachment especially when examining the impact of unresolved trauma of parents and the parent–child relationship (Main & Hesse, 1990; Ainsworth & Eichberg, 1991; Schuengel, Bakermans-Kranenburg, & Van Ijzendoorn, 1999). It appears that unresolved trauma may result in an inability of a mother to sensitively respond to the needs of her child. Many incarcerated mothers have unresolved trauma and loss issues and are unable to respond to the emotional and physical needs of their children. This study will explore trauma and attachment issues of mothers incarcerated in a minimum correctional facility for women.

Method

Women were voluntarily recruited to participate in a "family reunification" group by staff at a corrections center for women. A flyer was posted at the facility/prison, and interested women who met the inclusion criteria were informed by their counselor. Inclusion criteria for the group were as follows: (a) have at least one child or children; (b) child or children are involved with the child welfare system; (c) child or children in foster or kinship care placement; (d) family reunification was the permanency goal; (e) have regular planned parent–child visits; (f) a willingness to speak openly about problems including unresolved issues of trauma and attachment, problems that have impacted parenting, reasons for incarceration, relationship with child or children, etc.; and (g) an ability and commitment to maintain confidentiality. Counselors sent the names of women who voluntarily agreed to participate in the group to the assistant superintendent at the prison who contacted the group facilitators. All participants provided written informed consent for participation in the study. A Human Subjects Review Committee at the University of Washington approved the research protocol.

Participants

Twenty-eight women were in the family reunification group. The age range was 23 to 51 years, with a median age of 30.6 years. One woman reported that she had attended some college, six women had completed only high school, seven had their GED, two completed only the eleventh grade, one completed only the ninth grade, two completed only the seventh grade, one completed only the sixth grade, and four did not provide any information regarding their educational background. There were two African American women, two Latina women, one American Indian woman, and 23 White/European American women. There were five major reasons reported for incarceration: drugs (19 women), identity theft (six women), theft (seven women), fraud (four women), and burglary (two women).

Data collection

The AAI and the Trauma Attachment and Belief Scale (TABS) were administered. The AAI (George et al., 1984) is a semistructured, 1.5 to 2-hour protocol.

There are 18 questions. Each interview began by asking each participant to give a general description of her relationships to each parent and subsequently to give five adjectives that best represented the relationship with each parent. First, adjectives were given for the mother; participants were probed for specific memories of episodes that would support why each adjective was selected. This process was repeated for the father and any other significant attachment figure (e.g., stepmother, stepfather, etc.). The protocol continued by asking what the participant did when emotionally upset, physically hurt, or ill, and how the parents responded. Participants were asked about salient separations, possible experiences of rejection, threats regarding discipline, and any experience of abuse. Each participant was then asked about the effects of the aforementioned experiences on her adult personality, whether any of these experiences had a significant impact on development, and why the parents are believed to have engaged in the behavior discussed. The part of the AAI protocol that asks about experiences of loss of significant individuals because of death is very important. Whenever a respondent lost a significant individual in her life due to death the participant was probed regarding her reactions to the event, changes in feelings over time, and effects on adult personality. Finally, each participant was asked about the nature of her current relationship with parents and how experiences of being parented may have affected responses to her own child or children. The protocol was followed as written. All interviews were recorded via audiotape.

The TABS (Pearlman, 2003; Pearlman, Brock, & Hodgson, 2008) is a self-report instrument used to assess disrupted cognitive schemas (beliefs about self and about others) and need states associated with complex trauma exposure. Schemas in five areas that are sensitive to the effects of traumatic experiences were measured: safety, trust, esteem, intimacy, and control. Data yielded a total score and 10 subscale scores. There are 84 items on the TABS. Each participant was asked to rate on a 6-point Likert scale (1 = *Disagree strongly*, 6 = *Agree strongly*) the extent to which each statement matched her own beliefs. The items, which are face valid, fall in the "Easy" range on the Flesch Reading Ease Scale (Flesch, 1948, 1979) and are appropriate for anyone who can read at a third-grade level. The test scores have been demonstrated to be reliable for adults. In past samples, internal consistency and test-retest reliabilities for the TABS total score are good (0.96 and 0.75. respectively). The subscales are also reliable, with a median consistency estimate of 0.79 (range = 0.67 to 0.87) and a median test-retest reliability of 0.72 (range = 0.60 to 0.79) (Pearlman, 2003; Pearlman et al., 2008). Reliability was similar in this sample.

Data preparation and analysis

Average TABS raw scores were calculated for 10 variables: self-safety (the need to feel secure and reasonably invulnerable to harm inflicted by oneself or others); other-safety (the need to feel that cherished others are reasonably protected from harm inflicted by oneself or others); self-trust (the need to have confidence in one's own perceptions and judgment); other-trust (the need to depend or rely on others); self-esteem (the need to feel valuable and worthy of respect); other-esteem (the need to value and respect others); self-intimacy (the need to feel connected to one's own experience); other-intimacy (the need to feel connected to others); self-control (the need to manage one's feelings and behavior); and other control (the need to manage interpersonal situations). These scores were then converted to t-scores using data from the original normative sample.

The AAI is a semistructured 1.5- to 2-hour-long interview composed of questions that focus on childhood relationships with attachment figures, usually parents. The audiotaped responses were transcribed verbatim by a professional transcriptionist. Data were coded and classified by two coders who were extensively trained and certified at the University of California at Berkeley. The coders looked for independent evidence and counter evidence in each transcript and did cross-checking to enhance the validity of the data. Through analysis and coding of discourse, secure and insecure patterns of adult attachment were identified on the basis of three main classifications: autonomous, preoccupied, and dismissing. State of mind with respect to attachment is reflected in the AAI classifications. The meaning of each AAI classification is presented in Table 1. These classifications reflect differences in participants' mental representations based on differences in the organization of attachment experiences of each participant. The term for these mental representations is "internal working models" (Bowlby, 1969, p. 80).

Table 1. AAI Classifications.

Adult State of Mind with Respect to Attachment
Secure/autonomous (F)
Coherent, collaborative discourse, valuing of attachment, but seems objective regarding any particular event/relationship.
Description and evaluation of attachment-related experiences is consistent, whether experiences are favorable or unfavorable.
Dismissing (Ds)
Not coherent. Dismissing of attachment-related experiences and relationships. Normalizing ("excellent, very normal mother"), with generalized representations of history unsupported or actively contradicted by episodes recounted. Transcripts also tend to be excessively brief.
Preoccupied (E)
Not coherent. Preoccupied with or by past attachment relationships/experiences. Speaker appears angry, passive, or fearful. Sentences often long, grammatically entangled, or filled with vague usages ("dadadada," "and that"). Transcripts often excessively long.
Unresolved/disorganized (U)
During discussions of loss or abuse, individual shows striking lapse in the monitoring of reasoning or discourse. For example, individual may briefly indicate a belief that a dead person is still alive in the physical sense, or that this person was killed by a childhood thought. Individual may lapse into prolonged silence or eulogistic speech. The individual will ordinarily otherwise fit Ds, E, or F categories.

The summary of the adult attachment classifications is from Main et al. (1985) and from Main and Goldwyn (1994).

An internal working model is a conceptual framework of conscious and unconscious mental representations of attachment information for the purpose of understanding the world, self, and others (Bowlby, 1969; Main, Kaplan, & Cassidy, 1985).

Results

Mean TABS t-scores for participants are listed in Table 2. All scores reflect the participant's view of self in relation to others. The self-safety and other-safety t-scores were in the average range for the 28 participants (44 to 55). The self-trust and other-trust t-scores revealed that 10 participants were also in the average range (45 to 55) and 18 participants were in the high average range (56 to 59). t-scores for self-esteem and other-esteem, self-intimacy and other-intimacy, and self-control and other-control were in the average range (45 to 55). Interpretation of TABS t-score ranges are listed in Table 3.

The high-average score for the 18 participants in self-trust and other-trust seem to reflect a slightly negative view of self as well as a negative view of self in relation to others. Safety did not emerge as a distinct factor among the broader concepts of self and other. Evidence of safety as a primary experience is disrupted in direct as well as vicarious traumatization. Safety did not emerge as a distinct factor among the broader concepts of self and others. There was no sense of the abrogation of safety of either the self or other

Table 2. Average TABS t-scores for Family Reunification Group.

Psychological Needs	Mean	SD
Self-safety	44.8	14.1
Other-safety	53.3	12.3
Self-trust	56.6	17.1
Other-trust	51.9	13.6
Self-esteem	50.9	17.0
Other-esteem	54.8	11.7
Self-intimacy	51.9	13.6
Other-intimacy	55.8	12.0
Self-Control	54.9	7.8
Other Control	47.7	10.6

Table 3. Interpretation of TABS t-score Ranges.

T-Score	Interpretive Range
≤29	Extremely low (very little disruption)
30–39	Very low
49–44	Low average
45–55	Average
56–59	High average
60–69	Very high
≥70	Extremely high (substantial disruption)

From Pearlman (2003).

based on the average t-scores for self-safety and other-safety for participants in this study. Disrupted safety is a major feature of traumatic experience (Engelhard, Macklin, McNally, van der Hout, & Arntz, 2001; Iliffee & Steed, 2000; Overstreet & Braun, 2000; Pearlman & Saakvitne, 1995). There were no very high (60 to 69) or extremely high (.>70) scores for participants on any of the scales.

The AAI was used to have participants reflect on their childhood attachment experiences (primarily with parents) and assess possible impacts of these experiences on their personality and behavior. Classifications for participants were as follows: secure/autonomous ($n = 4$), dismissing ($n = 3$), preoccupied ($n = 6$), and unresolved/disorganized ($n = 15$). The narrative of participants classified as "secure/autonomous" (F) was coherent regardless of whether their experiences with their attachment figures were positive or negative. These participants answered questions with sufficient information but without excessively elaborating and were able to appropriately return the conversation to the group facilitator. Participants were classified as "dismissing" (Ds) when discourse seemed to be aimed at minimizing the discussion of attachment-related experiences. The narrative of these participants was not coherent because they are not internally consistent. Their descriptions of attachment figures were usually favorable to highly favorable; however, they did not provide supportive evidence for their positive representations and frequently contradicted themselves when providing their narratives. Participants classified as "preoccupied" (E) were unable to stay focused or to contain their responses, although the interview questions did stimulate their memories. Angry and lengthy responses were provided by participants in this category regarding childhood interactions with their attachment figures; their responses were often inappropriate and shifted to the present tense and/or discussion of the present relationship with attachment figures. Participants classified as "unresolved/disorganized" (U) had substantial lapses in monitoring of reasoning or discourse when discussing traumatic events such as experiences of major loss or abuse.

Discussion

This study focused on a small group of incarcerated mothers involved with the child welfare system and their unresolved issues of trauma and attachment. The findings suggest several issues that warrant discussion. These mothers are part of the increasingly large number of women who comprise the prison population today (Glaze & Maruschak, 2009; The Sentencing Project, 2015). The majority ($n = 19$) of the mothers in this study were incarcerated because of drug offenses. They had not committed major drug crimes but were often in a relationship with a man who was selling and/or using drugs, and usually in the wrong place at the wrong time, which resulted in their arrest and subsequent incarceration. The irony of this situation is that many of the men in their lives managed to escape arrest and incarceration and are still actively involved in the drug business. Once incarcerated for a drug offense the women in this study encountered the never-ending problem of trying to obtain treatment for their drug problems. Six women in the study are in a drug treatment program at the prison; however, the remaining 13 are on a waiting list for treatment.

According to Bowlby (1969), the quality of the early attachment relationship impacts relationships throughout the lifespan. Trauma has the capacity to shape one's physical, emotional, and intellectual development, especially when it is experienced in early childhood. Separation, loss, and grief were identified as traumatic experiences faced by mothers in this study. Most participants had insecure attachments and unresolved issues because of previous traumatic experiences. This finding is congruent with previous work regarding trauma exposure and unresolved issues of trauma (Berthelot et al., 2015; Iyengar et al., 2014; Murphy et al., 2014; Van Der Kolk et al., 1996).

The women classified as disorganized/disoriented (Main & Solomon, 1986, 1990) had early histories of abuse and neglect; early history of abuse and neglect is a format for disorganized/disorganized attachment (Carrion et al., 2001; Schore, 1994, 2003). Complex trauma was prevalent in the incarcerated mothers in this study. Several mothers had been abused and/or neglected by their primary attachment figures; this trauma was at the hands of parents whose responsibility was to love and protect them. Trauma in relation to a primary attachment figure tends to be more damaging than trauma in relation to a stranger. The earlier that trauma occurs in an individual's life, the greater is the damage, and the more severe the trauma, the greater is the potential for damage. Many of the unresolved trauma and attachment issues (i.e., separation, loss and grief, history of child abuse and/or neglect, etc.) resulted in drug use by mothers to alleviate the pain experienced from these issues (Harris, 2011, 2014). Incarcerated mothers expressed feelings of pain because of separation from their children and the lack of parent–child visits. They also experienced depression resulting from fear about having their parental rights terminated by the courts due to recommendation from child welfare workers and noncommunication from caregivers of their children. Grandmothers were the caregivers for many children of mothers in the study; these caregivers were also abusers during childhood of several mothers in the study.

There are important implications for policy, practice, and future research based on findings in this study. It is vital for social workers and other practitioners to assess adult attachment typology and unresolved issues of trauma and early history of child abuse and neglect. Unresolved issues of trauma and attachment cause difficulty for parents in building relationships and positive attachments with their children. The early attachment relationship is a substrate for subsequent relationships throughout the lifespan. Social workers and other practitioners need to be attuned to adverse effects on children when they are separated from parents because of incarceration. Best child welfare practice dictates that children must have regular visitation and communication with their primary attachment figure (i.e., mother and also their father if he is also incarcerated). If children are placed with relatives or in traditional foster care placements caregivers need to be informed about the significance of maintaining the parent–child relationship when a parent is incarcerated. Attachment disruptions can also be reduced when infants and/or young children are allowed to stay with their mothers in prison (Goslin, Byme, & Blanchard-Lewis, 2014; Harris, 1992). This residential arrangement allows social workers an opportunity to provide interventions to enhance the quality of the parent–child attachment relationship and should be encouraged as a best-practice for incarcerated pregnant women and for incarcerated women with very young children. Every member of society benefits when we value and support the mother–child attachment relationship when a mother is incarcerated, especially with the increase in births by pregnant women in prison.

Social workers need to maintain regular contact with their child's case manager or counselor at the prison where the child's mother or father is incarcerated. The social worker can gain knowledge regarding programs that are available to incarcerated parents and also inform the case manager or counselor about significant court dates and get approval for the incarcerated parent to participate from prison via telephone. The Adoption and Safe Families Act of 1997 (ASFA) has strict time guidelines for birth parents to make significant progress on the goals stipulated in the permanency plan (usually 12 months); however, judges have the authority to make exceptions. Because many parents have prison sentences that last longer than 12 months the child's social worker can petition the court for a longer time for a parent to achieve the goals in the permanency plan, especially when the goal is family reunification after a parent is released from prison.

Parents also need to be helped to understand the significance of language and the concept of time when communicating with their children. It is crucial for parents to always remember the child's age and developmental level in all communication. For example, the concept of time is very different for a 3-year-old toddler than for a 15-year-old adolescent.

Additional programs and services including clinical treatment are needed for incarcerated mothers and fathers in prison to prepare them for reentry into society and family reunification if reunification is the stated permanency goal. All services provided to incarcerated parents in prison should be family focused with an enhancement of the visiting environment for it to be sensitive to the needs of children. Previous research has shown that recidivism rates are lower for incarcerated women and men who have children and are reunited with these children after release from jail or prison. However, it is imperative for children of incarcerated parents and their families to have individualized services whenever their parents are released from prison. Incarcerated parents must be encouraged to stay in touch with their child's social worker about the permanency plan for their child and inform the child's social worker of their interest in family reunification when they are released from prison.

Several policies need to be reassessed and revised because they are not designed to support children of incarcerated parents, parents, and caregivers. These policies include the Anti-Drug Abuse Act of 1986 including the mandatory sentencing section; this law has resulted in the mass incarceration of many parents including mothers who have not committed major drug offenses. There is a need for drug policy reform. The also needs to be a reassessment of the Housing Opportunity Program Act of 1996 and the Quality Housing and Work Responsibility Act of 1998, especially the "One Strike" policy regarding public housing. Once an incarcerated mother and/or father is released from prison and submits an application for public housing many of these parents are immediately denied because of criminal records, especially if the record includes a drug offense.

Future research regarding issues of trauma and attachment need to include longitudinal studies that start in prison and are continued after incarcerated parents are released. A focus on intergenerational trauma and attachment is warranted in future research. Study samples must be large and include diverse populations, especially since the mass incarceration of men and women in this country results in a disproportionate number of people of color in jail and prison; this means that children of color are disproportionately represented in the child welfare system as a result of this mass incarceration (Harris, 2014).

Finally, there are several limitations of this study. The small sample size limited statistical power and the results cannot be generalized to the larger population of women who are incarcerated and involved with the child welfare system. The TABS was a self-report instrument, and there is the possibility that participants provided inaccurate responses to the test items.

Conclusion

The purpose of this study was to explore issues of unresolved trauma and attachment in a family reunification group of incarcerated mothers. The study highlighted the significance of the early attachment relationship and the impact of such on relationships across the lifespan. The study also illuminated the impact of unresolved traumatic experiences on adult attachment typology. Despite the limitations of the findings, the results provide a foundation for beginning to understand the relationship between unresolved trauma and attachment issues and the early attachment relationship when this relationship presents with a history of childhood abuse and neglect. This work extends previous work by focusing on incarcerated mothers. Although it is always crucial to provide services to children of incarcerated parents, it is imperative to include parents in service provision, especially incarcerated mothers who are the primary attachment figures and most often the caregivers for children. The best interest of the child should always be paramount in all policy, plans, and practice. Children are innocent and have not committed a crime; consequently, their right to an optimal mother–child relationship should be encouraged and supported, especially when mothers are incarcerated.

References

Ainsworth, M. D. S., Blehar, M. C., Waters, E., & Wall, S. (1978). *Patterns of attachment: A psychological study of the strange situation.* Hillsdale, NJ: Erlbaum.

Ainsworth, M. D. S., & Eichberg, C. G. (1991). Effects on infant-mother attachment of mother's unresolved loss of an attachment figure, or other traumatic experiences. In C. M. Parkes, J. Stevenson-Hinde, & P. Marris (Eds.), *Attachment across the life cycle* (pp. 160–183). New York, NY: Tavistock/Routledge.

Berthelot, N., Ensink, K., Bernazzani, O., Normandin, L., Luyten, P., & Fonagy, P. (2015). Intergenerational transmission of attachment in abused and neglected mothers: The role of reflective functioning. *Infant Mental Health Journal, 36*(2), 200–212. doi:10.1002/imhj.21499

Blatt, S. J., & Lerner, H. (1983). The psychological assessment of object representation. *Journal of Personality Assessment, 47*, 7–28. doi:10.1207/s15327752jpa4701_2

Bowlby, J. (1969). *Attachment and loss: Attachment* (Vol. 1). New York, NY: Basic Books.

Bowlby, J. (1973). *Attachment and loss: Attachment* (Vol. 2). New York, NY: Basic Books.

Bowlby, J. (1988). *A secure base: Parent-child attachment and healthy human development.* New York, NY: Basic Books.

Bowlby, J. (1989). *Secure and insecure attachment*. New York, NY: Basic Books.
Caffey, J. (1965). Significance of the history in the diagnosis of traumatic injury to children. *The Journal of Pediatrics, 67*, 1008–1014.
Caffey, J. (1972). On the theory and practice of shaking infants: Its potential residual effect of permanent brain damage and mental retardation. *American Journal of Diseases of Children, 124*, 161–169.
Campbell, C. S., & Robinson, J. W. (1997). Family and employment status associated with women's criminal behavior. *Psychological Reports, 80*, 307–314. doi:10.2466/pr0.1997.80.1.307
Carlen, P. (1998). *Sledgehammer: Women's imprisonment at the millennium*. Basingstoke, UK: MacMillan.
Carrion, V. G., Weems, C. F., Eliaz, S., Patwardham, A., Brown, W., & Ray, R. D. (2001). Attenuation of frontal asymmetry in pediatric posttraumatic stress disorder. *Biological Psychiatry, 50*, 943–951. doi:10.1016/S0006-3223(01)01218-5
Child Welfare League of America. (2001). *Alcohol, other drugs, and child welfare*. Washington, DC: Author.
Engelhard, I. M., Macklin, M. L., McNally, R. J., van der Hout, M. A., & Arntz, A. (2001). Emotion-and intrusion-based reasoning in Vietnam veterans with and without chronic posttraumatic stress disorder. *Behavior Research and Therapy, 39*, 1339–1348.
Erikson, E. (1968). *Identity: Youth and crisis*. New York, NY: W. W. Norton.
Flesch, R. (1948). A new read ability yardstick. *Journal of Applied Psychology, 32*(3), 221–233. doi:10.1037/h0057532
Flesch, R. (1979). *How to write plain English: Let's start with the formula*. Retrieved from http://pages.stern.nyu/≈wstarbick/wWriting/Flesch.htm
Fraiberg, S., Adelson, E., & Shapiro, V. (1975). Ghosts in the nursery: A psychoanalytic approach to the problem of impaired infant-mother relationships. *Journal of the American Academy of Child Psychiatry, 14*, 387–421. doi:10.1016/S0002-7138(09)61442-4
Freud, S. (1917). Mourning and melancholia. In *The Standard edition of the complete work psychological works of Sigmund Freud* (Vol. XIV, pp. 237–258). London, UK: Hogarth.
Freud, S. (1963). *Three essays on the theory of sexuality* (J. Strachey, Trans. & Ed.). New York, NY: Basic Books.
Frommer, E., & O'Shea, P. (1973). Antenatal identification of women likely to have problems in managing their infants. *British Journal of Psychology, 123*, 149–156. doi:10.1192/bjp.123.2.149
Frost, N. A., Greene, J., & Pranis, K. (2006). *Hard hit: The growth in the imprisonment of women, 1977-2004* (pp. 1–141). New York, NY: Women's Prison Association. Retrieved from htpp://www.wpaonline.org/institute/hardhit/HardHitReport4.pdf
George, C. (1984). *Individual differences in affective sensitivity: A study of five-year-olds and their parents*. Unpublished doctoral dissertation, University of California at Berkeley.
George, C., Kaplan, N., & Main, M. (1984). *Adult attachment interview protocol*. Unpublished manuscript, University of California at Berkeley, Berkeley, California.
George, C., & Solomon, J. (1996). Representational models of relationships: Links between caregiving and attachment. *Infant Mental Health Journal, 17*, 198–216. doi:10.1002/(ISSN)1097-0355
Glaze, L. E., & Maruschak, L. M. (2009). *Parents in prison and their minor children*. Washington, DC: Bureau of Justice Statistics.
Glaze, L. E., & Maruschak, L. M. (2011). *Parents in prison and their minor children*. Washington, DC: Bureau of Justice Statistics.
Goslin, L. S., Byme, M. W., & Blanchard-Lewis, B. (2014). Preschool outcomes of children who lived as infants in a prison nursery. *The Prison Journal, 94*(2), 139–158. doi:10.1177/0032885514524692

Gursansky, D., Harvey, J., McGrath, B., & O'Brien, B. (1998). *Who's minding the kids? Developing coordinated services for children whose mothers are imprisoned*. Adelaide, South Australia: Social Policy Research Group, University of South Australia.

Harris, J. (1992). Babies in prison. *Zero to Three, 13*, 17–21.

Harris, M. S. (2011). Adult attachment typology in a sample of high risk mothers. *Smith College Studies in Social Work, 81*(1), 41–61. doi:10.1080/00377317.2011.543043

Harris, M. S. (2014). *Racial disproportionality in child welfare* (pp. 1–23). New York, NY: Columbia University Press.

Harrison, P. M., & Beck, A. J. (2007). *Prisoners in 2005* (pp. 1–13). Washington, DC: U.S. Department of Justice, Office of Justice Programs.

Iliffee, G., & Steed, L. G. (2000). Exploring the counselor's experience of working with perpetrators and survivors of domestic violence. *Journal of Interpersonal Violence, 15*, 393–412.

Iyengar, U., Kim, S., Martinez, S., Fonagy, P., & Stratheam, L. (2014). Unresolved trauma in mothers' intergenerational effects and the role of reorganization. *Frontiers in Psychology, 5*, 1–9. doi:10.3389/fpsyg.2014.00966

LeFlore, L., & Holson, M. A. (1989). Perceived importance of parenting behaviors as reported by inmate mothers: An exploratory study. *Journal of Offender Counseling Services and Rehabilitation, 14*(1), 5–21. doi:10.1080/10509674.1989.9963921

Main, M., & Goldwyn, R. (1994). *Adult attachment rating and classification system*. Unpublished manuscript: Version 6.0, University of California at Berkeley, Berkeley, CA.

Main, M., & Hesse, E. (1990). Parents' unresolved traumatic experiences are related to infant disorganized status: Is frightened and/or frightening parental behavior the linking mechanism? In T. B. Brazelton & M. Yogman (Eds.), *Affective development in infancy* (pp. 95–124). Norwood, NJ: Ablex.

Main, M., Kaplan, N., & Cassidy, J. (1985). Security in infancy, childhood, and adulthood: A move to the level of representation. In J. Bretherton, & E. Waters (Eds.), Growing points of attachment theory and research. *Monographs of the Society for Research in Child Development, 50* (1–2), Serial No. 209, 66–104.

Main, M., & Solomon, J. (1986). Discovery of a new, insecure-disorganized/disoriented attachment pattern. In T. B. Brazelton, & M. Yogman (Eds.), *Affective development in infancy* (pp. 95–124). Norwood, NJ: Ablex.

Main, M., & Solomon, J. (1990). Procedures for identifying infants as disorganized/disoriented during the Ainsworth strange situation. In M. T. Greenberg, D. Cicchetti, & E. M. Cummings (Eds.), *Attachment in the preschool years: Theory, research, and intervention* (pp. 121–160). Chicago, IL: University of Chicago Press.

McGalliard, G. (2012, January 27). Record numbers of incarcerated mothers, bad news for women, children, communities. *Truthout*. Retrieved from www.truth-out.org/news/.../587/.record-numbers-of-incarcerated

Mukamal, D. A., & Samuels, P. N. (2002). Statutory limitations on civil rights of people with criminal records. *Fordham Urban Law Journal, 30*(5). Retrieved from htpp://ir.lawnet.fordham.edu/cgl/viewcontent.cgl?article – 18738context = ul

Murphy, A., Fernyhough, C., Fradley, E., & Tuckey, M. (2001). Rethinking maternal sensitivity: Mothers' comments on infants' mental processes predict security of attachment at 12 months. *Journal of Child Psychology and Psychiatry and Allied Disciplines, 42*, 637–648. doi:10.1111/1469-7610.00759

Murphy, A., Steele, M., Dube, S. R., Bale, J., Bonuck, K., Meisser, P., Goldman, H., & Steele, H. (2004). Adverse Childhood Experiences Questionnaire (ACEs) and Adult Attachment Interview (AAI): Implications for parent child relationships. *Child Abuse & Neglect, 38*(2), 224–233.

Overstreet, S., & Braun, S. (2000). Exposure to community violence and post-traumatic stress symptoms: Mediating factors. *American Journal of Orthopsychiatry, 70*(2), 263–271.

Pearlman, A. M., Brock, K. J., & Hodgson, S. T. (2008). Factor analysis of the trauma and attachment belief scale: A measure of cognitive schema disruption related to traumatic stress. *Journal of Psychological Trauma, 7*(3), 185–196. doi:10.1080/19322880802266813

Pearlman, L. A. (2003). *Trauma and attachment belief scale.* Los Angeles, CA: Western Psychological Services.

Pearlman, L. A., & Saakvitne, K. W. (1995). *Trauma and the therapist: Countertransference and vicarious traumatization in psychotherapy with incest survivors.* New York: W. W. Norton.

Philips, S. D., & Gleeson, J. P. (2007). *Children, families and the criminal justice system: A research brief.* Chicago, IL: Center for Social Policy and Research, University of Illinois, Chicago.

Riggs, S. A., Paulson, A., Tunnell, E., Sahl, G., Atkison, H., & Ross, C. A. (2007). Attachment, personality and psychopathology among adult inpatients: Self-reported romantic attachment style versus adult attachment interview states of mind. *Development and Psychopathology, 19,* 263–291. doi:10.1017/S0954579407070149

Rutter, M., & Madge, W. (1976). *Cycles of disadvantage: A review of research.* London, UK: Heinemann.

Rutter, Q. D., & Liddle, C. (1983). Parenting in two generations: Looking backwards and looking forward. In W. Madge (Ed.), *Families at risk* (pp. 60–98). London, UK: Heinemann.

Schore, A. N. (1994). *Affect regulation and the origin of the self: The neurobiology of emotional development.* Mahwah, NJ: Erlbaum.

Schore, A. N. (2001). Effects of a secure attachment relationship on right brain development, affect regulation, and infant mental health. *Infant Mental Health Journal, 22*(1–2), 7–66.

Schore, A. N. (2003). *Affect regulation and the repair of the self.* New York, NY: W. W. Norton.

Schuengel, C., Bakermans-Kranenburg, M. J., & Van Ijzendoorn, M. H. (1999). Frightening maternal behavior linking unresolved loss and disorganized infant attachment. *Journal of Consulting and Clinical Psychology, 67,* 54–63. doi:10.1037/0022-006X.67.1.54

Stovall-McClough, K. C., & Cloitre, M. (2006). Unresolved attachment, PTSD, and dissociation in women with childhood abuse histories. *Journal of Counseling and Clinical Psychology, 2,* 219–228.

Sykes, B., & Pettit, B. (2014). Mass incarceration, family complexity, and the reproduction of childhood disadvantage. *The Annals of the American Academy of Political and Social Science, 654*(1), 127–149. doi:10.1177/0002716214526345

The Sentencing Project. (2015). *Incarcerated women and girls* (pp. 1–5). Washington, DC: Author.

Van Der Kolk, B. A., Van Der Hart, O., & Marmar, C. R. (1996). Dissociation and information processing in posttraumatic stress disorder. In B. A. Van Der Kolk, A. C. McFarlane, & L. Weisaeth (Eds.), *Traumatic stress: The effects of overwhelming experience of mind, and society* (pp. 303–327). New York, NY: Guilford Press.

Winnicott, D. W. (1956). *Playing and reality.* London, UK: Tavistock.

Substance Use among Youth with Currently and Formerly Incarcerated Parents

Laurel Davis, PhD, and Rebecca J. Shlafer, PhD, MPH

> **ABSTRACT**
> Parental incarceration impacts millions of children in the United States and has important consequences for youths' adjustment. Children of incarcerated parents are at risk for a host of negative psychosocial outcomes, including substance abuse problems. Using data from a statewide survey of youth behavior, the effect of present and past parental incarceration on youths' report of their substance use behaviors was examined. Present and past parental incarceration was significantly associated with use of alcohol, tobacco, marijuana, and prescription drugs, as well as substance abuse and dependence. Implications for practice and research are discussed.

Mass incarceration, and its implications for children and families, is a growing concern for professionals across disciplines, including social work (Miller, 2006). According to the Bureau of Justice Statistics (BJS), there were more than 1.5 million people incarcerated in state and federal prisons in 2014 (Carson, 2015). In 2007, the last year for which BJS data are available, nearly 810,000 parents of 1.75 million children were incarcerated (Maruschak, Glaze, & Mumola, 2010). More recent data from the National Survey of Children's Health indicate that 7%, or 5 million children, have a history of parental incarceration (Murphey & Cooper, 2015).

Incarcerated parents report considerable socioeconomic and environmental risks (Glaze & Maruschak, 2008). There are profound disparities in incarceration rates by race (Carson, 2015), and as a result, there are a disproportionate number of children of color with incarcerated parents. Children living in poverty, those children whose parents have limited education, and children living in rural areas are also more likely to experience parental incarceration than their peers (Murphey & Cooper, 2015).

Substance abuse among incarcerated parents

The increase in the rate of parental incarceration during the past three decades (Glaze & Maruschak, 2008) is due in large part to increases in arrests and more severe penalties for drug-related offenses (Zhang, Maxwell, & Vaughn, 2009). In 2007, nearly 60% of incarcerated parents were serving time for drug-related offenses. Further, two out of three parents in state prisons met criteria for substance dependence or abuse, more than one-half (54%) reported using drugs in the month before their arrest, and more than one-third (34%) reported that during their childhoods, their parents or guardians had abused alcohol or drugs (Glaze & Maruschak, 2008). Youth who are exposed to parental substance abuse are more likely to abuse substances themselves (Clark, Cornelius, Kirisci, & Tarter, 2005), particularly when exposure occurs during the adolescent years (Biederman, Faraone, Monuteaux, & Feighner, 2000). The experience of risks such as these places youth with incarcerated parents at particularly high risk for intergenerational cycles of substance use and abuse and involvement with the criminal justice system.

Parental incarceration and youth outcomes

As an adverse childhood experience (ACE; Felitti et al., 1998), parental incarceration has consequences for children's social, emotional, behavioral, and physical health (Poehlmann & Eddy, 2010). Previous research has examined the potential consequences of parental incarceration for the next generation, including increased risk for antisocial behavior, mental health problems, and substance use (Huebner & Gustafson, 2007; Murray & Farrington, 2008; Murray, Janson, & Farrington, 2007; Murray, Loeber, & Pardini, 2012). For example, Dallaire and Aaron (2010) found that children who had a parent who was incarcerated in the past 2 years had higher levels of delinquency and were more likely to report experiencing family conflict and violence in their families than children who had experienced parental incarceration in the more distant past. Adolescents with incarcerated parents might also receive less monitoring from their caregivers, which can increase the likelihood that adolescents will engage in antisocial behavior such as aggression and substance use, particularly when they are spending time with peers who are engaging in such behaviors (Hanlon et al., 2005).

Studies have demonstrated links between parental incarceration and the substance use of youth. Murray and Farrington (2005) found that boys who were separated from a parent before age 10 because of incarceration were more likely to exhibit antisocial behaviors (including drug use and heavy drinking, among other indicators) in adolescence and adulthood compared with boys who experienced other types of childhood separations from parents. These findings remained significant even after controlling for parental criminality and other family risks. Likewise, Kinner, Alati, Najman, and Williams (2007) found that paternal imprisonment was associated with maternal reports of increased alcohol use among youth at age 14. However, these associations became nonsignificant when a variety of family characteristics were controlled (e.g., socioeconomic status, maternal mental health, maternal substance use).

Adolescence as a sensitive period

Adolescence may be a particularly sensitive period for the onset of behavior problems and substance use (Chassin, Sher, Hussong, & Curran, 2013). Adolescence is a time when the brain is still developing and risk-taking is normative (Casey & Jones, 2010), including some experimentation with substance use. However, substance use that begins in the adolescent period is associated with higher rates of dependence, disruptive behaviors, and major depression in adulthood (Clark, Kirisci, & Tarter, 1998). Early initiation of substances and frequent substance use may make adolescents more likely to become involved in the juvenile justice system and subsequently the adult criminal justice system, contributing to an intergenerational cycle of incarceration (Wakefield & Uggen, 2010). Studies have placed estimates of substance use disorders in juvenile justice populations as high as 62% (Aarons, Brown, Hough, Garland, & Wood, 2001). For example, in a sample of young people in a juvenile detention center in Cook County, IL, Teplin and colleagues (Teplin, Abram, McClelland, Dulcan, & Mericle, 2002) found that half of males and nearly half of females had a substance use disorder. Further, substance use predicts recidivism in adolescent populations, even after controlling for sociodemographic variables and prior delinquency (Stoolmiller & Blechman, 2005). In fact, onset of a substance use disorder by the age 16 is associated with a fourfold greater risk of incarceration for substance-related offenses in adulthood, compared with those with no disorder (Slade et al., 2008).

Combined, the high rates of substance abuse among incarcerated parents (Glaze & Maruschak, 2008), previous research linking parental incarceration with adverse outcomes in the next generation, and the developmental salience of substance use in adolescence make substance use among youth with incarcerated parents an important area for scientific inquiry. As such, this study examines substance use in youth with currently and formerly incarcerated parents, compared with children with no history of parental incarceration.

Research questions

Based on previous research, we expect that children of currently incarcerated parents will exhibit higher rates of substance use than those with formerly incarcerated parents and that both groups will report more substance use than children with no experience of parental incarceration, after controlling for demographic characteristics and household substance abuse.

Method

Data source

Data for this study were drawn from the 2013 Minnesota Student Survey (MSS; Minnesota Department of Education, 2015). The MSS is administered every 3 years to all fifth-, eighth-, ninth-, and eleventh-grade students in Minnesota. It includes self-reported data from young people on use of alcohol, tobacco, and other drugs. Student participation is voluntary and all surveys are completely anonymous; no identifying information is collected. School districts are required to follow federal laws regarding parental notification, as required by the Family Educational Rights and Privacy Act and the Protection of Pupil Rights Amendment. In 2013, 84% of public school districts and 71% of eighth-graders, 69% of ninth-graders, and 62% of eleventh-graders participated (Minnesota Department of Education, 2015). In 2013, the most recent year for which data are available, the survey was completed by 42,841 students in eighth grade, 42,381 students in ninth grade, and 36,958 students in eleventh grade ($N = 122,180$). For the first time in 2013, youth were asked to report whether they have a parent or guardian who has even been in jail or prison.

Participants

Participants in this study were 122,180 children in public schools in the state of Minnesota who provided data on the 2013 MSS survey. On average, youth were 14.87 years old ($SD = 1.34$, range = 12 to 19 years), and half of the youth in the sample (50.2%, $n = 61,341$) were boys. Reflecting the demographics of the state of Minnesota as a whole, most of the youth in the sample (72.9%) identified as non-Hispanic White.

Measures

Dependent variables

Dependent variables in this study included: early alcohol initiation, recent alcohol use, binge drinking, tobacco use, lifetime marijuana use, recreational use of prescription drugs, substance abuse or dependence, and treatment for drug or alcohol problems.

Early alcohol initiation. Students in ninth and eleventh grades only were asked, "How old were you when you had your first drink of an alcoholic beverage such as beer, wine, wine coolers, and liquor, other than a few sips?" Response choices ranged from 10 to 17 years, or "I have never had a drink of alcohol other than a few sips." Youth who reported drinking at 12 years or younger were coded "1"; all other students were coded "0." Full text of the survey items is available from the authors on request.

Recent alcohol use. Students were asked, "During the last 30 days, on how many days did you drink one or more drinks of an alcoholic beverage?" There were seven response choices, ranging from 0 to 30 days. Students who endorsed any use of alcohol in the 30-day period were coded "1"; students who endorsed 0 days were coded "0."

Binge drinking. Binge drinking was measured by combining two items: the number of drinking occasions in the past 12 months and average alcohol consumption on those occasions. Students were asked, "If you drink beer/wine/wine coolers/liquor, generally how much (if any) do you drink at one time?" Response options ranged from one to five drinks, or "I don't drink beer/wine/wine coolers/liquor." Students were also asked, "During the last 12 months, on how many occasions (if any) have you had alcoholic beverages to drink?" Response options ranged from 0–40 or more. Students who endorsed drinking an average of five or more drinks on 10 or more occasions in the past year were coded "1"; otherwise they were coded "0."

Tobacco use. Frequent use of tobacco was measured with three items. Students were asked the following three questions: "During the last 30 days, on how many days did you smoke a cigarette?" "During the last 30 days, on how many days did you smoke cigars, cigarillos, or little cigars?" and "During the last 30 days, on how many days did you use chewing tobacco, snuff, or dip?" For all three questions, response options ranged from 0 to 30 days. Students who endorsed use of any type of tobacco on 20 or more days were coded "1"; otherwise they were coded "0."

Lifetime marijuana use. Students in ninth and eleventh grades were asked, "How old were you when you tried marijuana (pot, weed) or hashish (hash, hash oil) for the first time?" Answers ranged from 10 to 17 years or "I have never used tried marijuana or hashish." Students who endorsed any use of marijuana, regardless of the age of use, were coded "1"; otherwise they were coded "0."

Recreational use of prescription drugs. Students were asked, "During the last 30 days, on how many days did you use prescription drugs not prescribed for you?" Response choices ranged from 0 to 30 days. Students who endorsed using prescription drugs on 1 or more days were coded "1"; otherwise they were coded "0."

Substance abuse or dependence. The MSS includes 13 questions that represent the *Diagnostic and Statistical Manual of Mental Disorders, Fourth*

Edition (DSM–4; First, 1994) criteria for a substance use disorder. Students who endorsed no use in the past 12 months were coded "not applicable" ($n = 76{,}667$) and excluded from this analysis.

Five items measure the four DSM-4 criteria for substance abuse: (1) "During the last 12 months, how many times have you missed work or school, or neglected other major responsibilities because of alcohol or drug use?" (2) "During the last 12 months, how many how many times have you driven a motor vehicle while using alcohol or drugs?" (3) During the last 12 months, how many times has alcohol or drug use caused you problems with the law?" (4A) During the last 12 months, have you continued to use alcohol or drugs even though you knew it was hurting your relationships with friends or family?" or (4B) "During the last 12 months, how many times have you hit someone or become violent after using alcohol or drugs?" For items 1, 2, 3, and 4B, response options ranged from zero to three times. For item 4A, response options were "Yes" or "No." Any student who reported a positive response on at least one criterion was coded "1"; otherwise they were coded as "0."

Seven items measured the seven DSM-4 criteria for substance dependence: (1) "During the last 12 months have you found that you had to use a lot more alcohol or drugs than before to get the same effect?" (2) "During the last 12 months, how many times have you used more alcohol or drugs than you intended to?" (3) "During the last 12 months, have you tried to cut down on your use of alcohol or drugs but couldn't?" (4) "During the last 12 months, how many times have you spent all or most of the day using alcohol or drugs, or getting over their effects?" (5) "During the last 12 months, how many times have you given up important social or recreational activities like sports or being with friends or relatives to use alcohol or drugs or to get over their effects?" (6A) "During the last 12 months, how many times has alcohol or drug use left you feeling depressed, agitated, paranoid, or unable to concentrate?" or (6B) "During the last 12 months, how many times have you used so much alcohol or other drugs that the next day you could not remember what you had said or done?" For items 1 and 4, response options were "Yes" or "No." For all other items, response options ranged from zero to three times. Any student who reported a positive response on at least three of those criteria was coded "1"; otherwise, they were coded as "0." The substance abuse and dependence scales were combined into a single outcome variable; students who met either the abuse or dependence criteria were coded "1"; otherwise, they were coded "0."

Treatment for drug or alcohol problems. Students were asked, "Have you ever been treated for an alcohol or drug problem? (Mark ALL that apply)." Response options were "No," "Less, during the last year," or "Yes, more than a year ago." Students who endorsed receiving treatment for a drug or alcohol use problem at any time were coded "1"; otherwise, they were coded "0." Treatment for alcohol or drug problems is relevant only to those students who reported using substances; therefore, students who endorsed no use of any substance in the past 12 months were coded "not applicable" (*n* = 76,667) and excluded from this analysis.

Independent variables

Independent variables were current or former experience of parental incarceration, gender, age, poverty, race and ethnicity, urbanicity, and exposure to household substance abuse.

Parental incarceration. Parental incarceration was assessed with one item: "Have any of your parents or guardians ever been in jail or prison? (Mark ALL that apply)." Answer choices were "None of my parents or guardians has ever been in jail or prison," "Yes, I have a parent or guardian in jail or prison right now," and "Yes, I have a parent or guardian in jail or prison in the past." Most respondents (77.5%) indicated no experience of parental incarceration, 13% indicated that a parent was incarcerated in the past, and 1.8% indicated that a parent was currently incarcerated; 7.7% of responses were missing. There were a small number of children (*n* = 579; 0.47%) who reported they had a currently and formerly incarcerated parent; these children were included in the currently incarcerated parent category. Thus, parental incarceration was a three-level variable coded "0" = "No experience of parental incarceration," "1" = "Formerly incarcerated parent," and "2" = "Currently incarcerated parent."

Gender. Gender was assessed with one item. Students were asked to report their gender, with response options of "male" or "female." Males were coded "0"; females were coded "1".

Age. Age was assessed with one item. Students were asked, "How old are you?" Response options ranged from 11 years to 21 years or older. No students reported being 11 years or younger or 21 years or older. Thus, age ranged from 12 to 19 years.

Poverty. On the basis of previous research with these data set (Gower, McMorris, & Eisenberg, 2015), poverty status was assessed with three items: "Do you currently get free or reduced-price lunch at school?" "During the last 30 days, have you had to skip meals because your family did not have enough money to buy food?" and "During the past 12 months, have you stayed in a shelter, somewhere not intended as a place to live, or someone else's home because you had no other place to stay?" Respondents who endorsed any one of these items were coded "1"; otherwise, they were coded "0."

Race and ethnicity. Race and ethnicity were measured with six items. Students were asked whether they identify with any of the following racial or ethnic groups: Hispanic or Latino/a; American Indian or Alaskan Native; Asian; Black, African, or African American; Native Hawaiian or Other Pacific Islander; White. We would like to be able to examine racial and ethnic groups separately, given potential differential outcomes. However, because most students reported they were non-Hispanic White, sample sizes for the other races and ethnicities were relatively small. Further, although our overall sample is large, it includes just 2,202 children with a currently incarcerated parent. Logistic regression requires that no cells contain sparse data, which becomes increasingly untenable as the number of covariates increases. Given these considerations, race and ethnicity were treated dichotomously. Students were coded "0" if they endorsed only "White"; otherwise, they were coded "1."

Urbanicity. Students in schools located in the seven-county major metropolitan area were coded "0"; students in schools outside the metropolitan area were coded "1."

Exposure to household substance abuse. Adult household substance abuse was measured with two items: "Do you live with anyone who drinks too much alcohol?" and "Do you live with anyone who uses illegal drugs or abuses prescription drugs?" Response options for both items were "Yes" or "No." Students who reported "Yes" for either question were coded "1"; students who responded "No" to both items were coded "0." A greater proportion of youth with currently (59%) and formerly (47%) incarcerated parents reported living with someone who abuses substances than youth with no experience of parental incarceration (33%).

Data analysis

Analyses were conducted with the use of SPSS v. 23. Logistic regression models were used to examine differences in substance use by parental incarceration status, while controlling for gender, age, poverty, race/ethnicity, urbanicity, and exposure to household substance use. Separate models were run for each measure of substance use.

Missing data

Overall, the level of missing data was small, ranging from complete data for gender to 7.7% for parental incarceration. However, the sample sizes were different among the outcomes examined. Two of the outcomes—age of initiation of alcohol use and marijuana use—were asked only of the ninth- and eleventh-grade students. Some outcomes, such as substance abuse or dependence or treatment for drug or alcohol problems, are relevant only for those youth who reported using substances. Sample sizes for all outcomes are reported in Table 1.

Table 1. Descriptive Statistics by Incarceration Status.

	n	Full Sample Mean (SD)/%	0 = None Mean (SD)/%	1 = Former Mean (SD)/%	2 = Current Mean (SD)/%
Age (yr)	121,919	14.9 (1.34)	14.9 (1.34)	14.8 (1.31)	14.8 (1.29)
Gender (1 = female)	122,180	49.8	50.3	53.7	48.2
Poverty (1 = at least 1 risk)	121,954	30.9	23.7	59.7	74.8
Race/ethnicity (1 = not white)	120,715	26.3	21.6	38.6	54.6
Urbanicity (1 = non-metro area)	122,180	46.9	46.9	55.5	50.1
Household substance abuse (1 = yes)	113,452	13.5	9.7	32.3	38.1
Early alcohol initiation (1 = yes)	72,285	37.7	35.7	48.5	46.7
Recent alcohol use (1 = yes)	112,521	16.8	14.3	28.4	36.7
Binge drinking (1 = yes)	111,168	2.4	1.9	4.4	6.3
Frequent tobacco use (1 = yes)	113,349	3.1	2.1	7.1	14.6
Lifetime marijuana use (1 = yes)	72,439	23.7	19.5	44.3	58.1
Use of prescription drugs (1 = yes)	111,344	5.3	3.9	11.5	21.7
Abuse or dependence (1 = yes)	27,941	37.5	33.4	46.7	58.9
Drug or alcohol treatment (1 = yes)	42,903	5.7	3.9	9.9	22.4

Results

More than 16% of the youths surveyed endorsed use of alcohol in the past 30 days. Early alcohol initiation (use at age 12 or earlier) was endorsed by 37.7% of students in ninth and eleventh grades, and binge drinking was reported by 2.4% of all youth in the sample. More than 23% of youth in ninth and eleventh grades endorsed prior use of marijuana, and just over 5% of all students endorsed misuse of prescription drugs. Of the students who reported any use of drugs or alcohol ($n = 45,513$, or 37.3% of all students), 35.3% met the DSM criteria for substance abuse or dependence disorder; however, fewer than 6% of youth who reported substance use had received treatment. About 3% of youth reported being regular users of tobacco products. Across all the outcomes, adolescents with currently and formerly incarcerated parents exhibited higher rates of problems than children with no history of parental incarceration. Descriptive statistics by incarceration group can be found in Table 1.

Logistic regression analyses, controlling for demographic characteristics and household substance use, supported the hypothesis that children of currently and formerly incarcerated parents were more likely to use and abuse alcohol, tobacco, and other drugs than were children with no experience of parental incarceration. For seven of the eight outcomes, children of currently incarcerated parents exhibited the highest risk, followed by children of formerly incarcerated parents. Adjusted odds ratios are presented in Table 2.

Compared with children with no experience of parental incarceration, adolescents with formerly incarcerated parents were 1.5 times as likely to report trying alcohol at age 12 or younger. They were about twice as likely to report prescription drug use, binge drinking, and recent alcohol consumption. Youth with a formerly incarcerated parent were more than twice as likely to report using tobacco and marijuana and were 1.5 times as likely to meet DSM criteria for substance abuse or dependence.

Table 2. Adjusted Odds Ratios from Logistic Regression Models.

	B	SEB	OR (95% CI)
Early alcohol initiation			
Incarceration (ref = none)			
Formerly	0.41***	0.03	1.51 (1.44–1.58)
Currently	0.32***	0.06	1.38 (1.22–1.55)
Recent alcohol use			
Incarceration (ref = none)			
Formerly	0.62***	0.02	1.86 (1.78–1.95)
Currently	1.00***	0.05	2.73 (2.47–3.01)
Binge drinking			
Incarceration (ref = none)			
Formerly	0.66***	0.05	1.93 (1.74–2.14)
Currently	1.04***	0.10	2.82 (2.30–3.46)
Tobacco use			
Incarceration (ref = none)			
Formerly	0.88***	0.04	2.41 (2.21–2.63)
Currently	1.67***	0.08	5.33 (4.60–6.18)
Marijuana use			
Incarceration (ref = none)			
Formerly	0.93***	0.03	2.54 (2.41–2.70)
Currently	1.40***	0.06	4.06 (3.59–4.59)
Prescription drug abuse			
Incarceration (ref = none)			
Formerly	0.72***	0.04	2.05 (1.91–2.19)
Currently	1.39***	0.06	4.03 (3.57–4.55)
Abuse or dependence on drugs or alcohol			
Incarceration (ref = none)			
Formerly	0.43***	0.03	1.53 (1.44–1.63)
Currently	0.86***	0.07	2.37 (2.06–2.73)
Treatment for drug or alcohol abuse			
Incarceration (ref = none)			
Formerly	0.59***	0.05	1.81 (1.63–2.01)
Currently	1.26***	0.08	3.90 (3.33–4.56)

Note: Statistics reported in this table have been adjusted for adolescent age, gender, race/ethnicity, exposure to poverty, urbanicity, and household substance use.
***$p < .001$.

When compared with children with no history of parental incarceration, children of currently incarcerated parents were more likely to report using alcohol before the age of 12. They were more than twice as likely to report recent alcohol use and binge drinking, four times as likely to report use of marijuana or prescription drugs and more than five times as likely to report using tobacco products. They were 2.4 times as likely to meet DSM criteria for substance abuse or dependence, and 3.9 times as likely to have received treatment for drug or alcohol abuse.

Discussion

Results of this study demonstrated that youth with currently and formerly incarcerated parents were more likely to report substance use and abuse compared with youth who have never experienced the incarceration of a parent.

Additionally, youth with currently incarcerated parents fared worse than their peers with a history of parental incarceration on nearly every indicator. The higher rates of substance use and abuse among youth with incarcerated parents have important implications for youth well-being within multiple domains of functioning and across the lifespan. Longitudinal research shows that early alcohol and drug use predicts failure to complete high school, even after controlling for other risk factors (McCluskey, Krohn, Lizotte, & Rodriguez, 2002). High rates of substance use and abuse may be one mechanism by which social inequality is systematically transmitted across generations, including in families with incarcerated parents (Wakefield & Uggen, 2010).

There are at least four possible mechanisms by which parental incarceration may be linked to adolescents' substance use. The first mechanism, which parallels the work of Turney and Haskins (2014) on academic outcomes among young children with incarcerated parents, suggests that a child's separation from her parent as a result of the parent's incarceration may be a traumatic experience. Arditti (2012) documented symptoms of posttraumatic stress in children with incarcerated mothers, including depression, trouble sleeping, and concentration problems. Among adolescents with limited social support and poor coping skills, distress resulting from trauma could lead to alcohol and drug use as a coping behavior (Travis, McBride, & Solomon, 2005).

A second possible mechanism emphasizes strain to the family system as a result of the parent's incarceration, through the loss of income, disruption in parenting roles, housing mobility, and conflict in the coparenting relationship (Foster & Hagan, 2009). This strain may compromise children's adjustment and consequently increase their risk for antisocial behavior, including substance use and abuse (Agnew, 1992).

A third potential mechanism involves genetic risk. Incarcerated parents may have poor impulse control (Meldrum, Young, & Lehmann, 2015), and many have a history of addiction, which may have ultimately contributed to their incarcerations (Glaze & Maruschak, 2008). As such, many adolescents with incarcerated parents may be genetically predisposed to substance use disorders.

A fourth mechanism concerns adolescents' environmental exposures. Rates of substance use and abuse are higher in inmate populations than in the general public. Children with incarcerated parents may be more likely to have lived in a household where someone abused drugs or alcohol, as was indeed the case in our sample. Exposure to a parent's substance abuse is a potent risk factor for children's substance abuse (Biederman et al., 2000). It is possible that parental drug and alcohol abuse, which is related to parental incarceration, is the underlying causal mechanism rather than incarceration itself.

These mechanisms for the transmission of risk are likely overlapping and interconnected. Although the cross-sectional nature of the data limit our ability to draw casual inferences or empirically test these mechanisms, the results point to valuable areas for future inquiry and existing large-scale data

Implications for social work practice

These findings point professionals to potential areas for prevention and intervention, including the adaptation of evidence-based programs to meet specific needs of youth affected by a parent's incarceration. An example of a promising approach for youth substance use is the cognitive-behavioral Families Facing the Future (FFF; formerly known as Focus on Families) program (University of Washington Social Development Research Group, n.d.). FFF was developed for parents receiving methadone treatment and their children. The program aims to (a) reduce parents' use of illegal drugs and (b) to reduce their children's risk factors for future drug use, while also promoting protective factors (e.g., family communication). Research has demonstrated initial positive effects on parent and youth outcomes, including increased relapse prevention skills and increased self-efficacy skills, which were linked to reductions in substance use and family conflict (Catalano, Gainey, Fleming, Haggerty, & Johnson, 1999). At 2-year follow-up, children in FFF reported less substance use and fewer behavior problems (Bry, Catalano, Kumpfer, Lochman, & Szapocznik, 1998). Although FFF offers a promising approach, to the best of our knowledge, the feasibility of administering FFF with currently incarcerated parents has not yet been established, and outcomes with this population are yet unknown.

Limitations

The current study has several limitations. First, the study relied exclusively on youths' self-reports of their substance use, abuse, and treatment. Prior research has found self-reports of substance use to have good reliability (Johnson & Mott, 2001) and moderate validity (Williams & Nowatzki, 2005). Combining youths' self-reports with parent reports, peer reports, and/or juvenile court records would strengthen future studies. A second limitation relates to potential selection effects. Although all school districts in the state were invited and encouraged to participate, two large public school districts in urban areas opted out. Given the concentration of social disadvantage and crime in urban areas (Bobo, 2009; Rodriguez, 2013), we suspect that results presented here likely underrepresent the true number of youth who have experienced a parent's incarceration. Similarly, the Minnesota Student Survey only surveys youth currently attending school. Substance abuse may contribute to academic difficulties and school failure and/or lead to placements outside of school (e.g., in patient treatment programs); thus, some students with substance use problems may have not been in school and thus not included in this sample. Furthermore, youth who drop out of school may be disproportionally affected by parental incarceration. Issues such as these may have impacted our estimates on the relation between parental incarceration on youths' substance use and abuse.

Finally, the 2013 Minnesota Student Survey included only a single item about the incarceration of a parent or guardian. No information was collected about which parent or guardian was incarcerated, the circumstances of the incarceration, or the timing, frequency, or duration of the parent's incarceration. Effects may vary depending on the child's developmental capacities at the time the parent is incarcerated and by the frequency of incarceration (Shlafer & Poehlmann, 2010). The youth's caregiver(s) before, during, and after the parent's incarceration, disruptions in the home environment due to the incarceration, and the incarcerated parent's role upon release are examples of important factors to assess in future research.

Conclusions

Despite these limitations, this study provides important information about the use of alcohol, tobacco, and other drugs among youth with currently and formerly incarcerated parents compared with those who have not had these experiences. Results from this study indicate that parental incarceration is a potentially potent risk factor for adolescents' substance use and abuse. Given the long-term consequences of early substance use, and especially early frequent and heavy use, this study has important implications for professionals working with youth with an incarcerated parent.

Acknowledgments

The authors wish to thank the members of the Minnesota Strengthening Families Affected by Incarceration Collaborative for their early guidance identifying youth outcomes of particular interest to community stakeholders

Funding

This project was supported by the Health Resources and Services Administration (HRSA) of the U.S. Department of Health and Human Services (HHS) under the National Research Service Award (NRSA) in Primary Medical Care (T32HP22239; PI: Borowsky) and the National Institutes of Health (NIH) Clinical and Translational Science Institute at the University of Minnesota (UL1TR000114; PI: Blazer). The content and conclusions are those of the authors and should not be construed as the official position or policy of, nor should any endorsements be inferred by HRSA, HHS, NIH, or the U.S. Government.

References

Aarons, G. A., Brown, S. A., Hough, R. L., Garland, A. F., & Wood, P. A. (2001). Prevalence of adolescent substance use disorders across five sectors of care. *Journal of the American Academy of Child & Adolescent Psychiatry, 40*(4), 419–426. doi:10.1097/00004583-200104000-00010

Agnew, R. (1992). Foundation for a general strain theory of crime and delinquency. *Criminology, 30*(1), 47–88. doi:10.1111/j.1745-9125.1992.tb01093.x

Arditti, J. (2012). Child trauma within the context of parental incarceration: A family process perspective. *Journal of Family Theory & Review, 4*(3), 181–219. doi:10.1111/j.1756-2589.2012.00128.x

Biederman, J., Faraone, S. V., Monuteaux, M. C., & Feighner, J. A. (2000). Patterns of alcohol and drug use in adolescents can be predicted by parental substance use disorders. *Pediatrics, 106*(4), 792–797. doi:10.1542/peds.106.4.792

Bobo, L. D. (2009). Crime, urban poverty, and social science. *Du Bois Review: Social Science Research on Race, 6*, 273–278. doi:10.10170S1742058X0999021X

Bry, B. H., Catalano, R. F., Kumpfer, K. L., Lochman, J. E., & Szapocznik, J. (1998). Scientific findings from famliy prevention intervention research. In R. S. Ashery, E. B. Robertson, & K. L. Kumpfe (Eds.), *Drug Abuse Prevention Through Family Interventions* (pp. 103–129). Collingdale, PA: DIANE Publishing.

Carson, E. (2015). *Prisoners in 2014 (NCJ 248955)*. (L. McConnell & J. Thomas, Eds.). Washington, DC: U. S. Department of Justice, Bureau of Justice Statistics.

Casey, B. J., & Jones, R. M. (2010). Neurobiology of the adolescent brain and behavior: Implications for substance use disorders. *Journal of the American Academy of Child and Adolescent Psychiatry, 49*(12), 1189–1201. doi:10.1016/j.jaac.2010.08.017

Catalano, R. F., Gainey, R. R., Fleming, C. B., Haggerty, K. P., & Johnson, N. O. (1999). An experimental intervention with families of substance abusers: One-year follow-up of the focus on families project. *Addiction, 94*(2), 241–254. doi:10.1046/j.1360-0443.1999.9422418.x

Chassin, L., Sher, K. J., Hussong, A., & Curran, P. (2013). The developmental psychopathology of alcohol use and alcohol disorders: Research achievements and future directions. *Development and Psychopathology, 25*, 1567–1584. doi:10.1017/S0954579413000771.The

Clark, D. B., Cornelius, J. R., Kirisci, L., & Tarter, R. E. (2005). Childhood risk categories for adolescent substance involvement: A general liability typology. *Drug and Alcohol Dependence, 77*, 13–21. doi:10.1016/j.drugalcdep.2004.06.008

Clark, D. B., Kirisci, L., & Tarter, R. E. (1998). Adolescent versus adult onset and the development of substance use disorders in males. *Drug and Alcohol Dependence, 49*(2), 115–121. doi:10.1016/S0376-8716(97)00154-3

Dallaire, D. H., & Aaron, L. (2010). Middle childhood: Family, school, and peer contexts for children affected by parental incarceration. In J. M. Eddy, & J. Poehlmann (Eds.), *Children of incarcerated parents: A handbook for researchers and practitioners* (pp. 101–120). Washington, DC: Urban Institute Press.

Felitti, V. J., Anda, R. F., Nordenberg, D., Williamson, D. F., Spitz, A. M., Edwards, V., ... Marks, J. S. (1998). Relationship of childhood abuse and household dysfunction to many of the leading causes of death in adults: The Adverse Childhood Experiences (ACE) Study. *American Journal of Preventive Medicine, 14*(4), 245–258. doi:10.1016/S0749-3797(98)00017-8

First, M. B. (1994). *Diagnostic and statistical manual of mental disorders. DSM IV-4th edition.* Washington, DC: American Psychological Association.

Foster, H., & Hagan, J. (2009). The mass incarceration of parents in America: Issues of race/ethnicity, collateral damage to children, and prisoner reentry. *The ANNALS of the American Academy of Political and Social Science, 623*(1), 179–194. doi:10.1177/0002716208331123

Glaze, L. E., & Maruschak, L. L. M. (2008). *Parents in prison and their minor children.* Washington, DC: U.S. Department of Justice, Bureau of Justice Statistics. Retrieved from http://www.ncjrs.gov/App/abstractdb/AbstractDBDetails.aspx?id=244893

Gower, A. L., McMorris, B. J., & Eisenberg, M. E. (2015). School-level contextual predictors of bullying and harassment experiences among adolescents. *Social Science & Medicine, 147*, 47–53. doi:10.1016/j.socscimed.2015.10.036

Hanlon, T. E., Blatchley, R. J., Bennett-Sears, T., O'Grady, K. E., Rose, M., & Callaman, J. M. (2005). Vulnerability of children of incarcerated addict mothers: Implications for preventive intervention. *Children and Youth Services Review, 27*(1), 67–84. doi:10.1016/j.childyouth.2004.07.004

Harris, K. M., Halpern, C. T., Whitsel, E., Hussey, J., Tabor, J., Entzel, P., & Udry, J. R. (2009). *The national longitudinal study of adolescent health: Research design.* Chapel Hill, NC: Carolina Population Center, University of North Carolina-Chapel Hill. Retrieved from http://www.icpsr.umich.edu/icpsrweb/DSDR/studies/27021/version/9

Huebner, B. M., & Gustafson, R. (2007). The effect of maternal incarceration on adult offspring involvement in the criminal justice system. *Journal of Criminal Justice, 35*(3), 283–296. doi:10.1016/j.jcrimjus.2007.03.005

Johnson, T. P., & Mott, J. A. (2001). The reliability of self reported age of onset of tobacco, alcohol and illicit drug use. *Addiction, 96*(8), 1187–1198. doi:10.1080/09652140120060770

Kinner, S. A., Alati, R., Najman, J. M., & Williams, G. M. (2007). Do paternal arrest and imprisonment lead to child behaviour problems and substance use? A longitudinal analysis. *Journal of Child Psychology and Psychiatry, 48*(11), 1148–1156. doi:10.1111/j.1469-7610.2007.01785.x

Maruschak, L. M., Glaze, L. E., & Mumola, C. J. (2010). Incarcerated Parents and their Children. In J. M. Eddy, & J. Poehlmann (Eds.), *Children of incarcerated parents: A handbook for researchers and practitioners* (pp. 33–51). Washington, DC: Urban Institute Press.

McCluskey, C. P., Krohn, M. D., Lizotte, A. J., & Rodriguez, M. L. (2002). Early substance use and school achievement: An examination of Latino, White, and African American youth. *Journal of Drug Issues, 32*(3), 921–943. doi:10.1177/002204260203200313

Meldrum, R. C., Young, J. T. N., & Lehmann, P. S. (2015). Parental low self-control, parental socialization, young adult low self-control, and offending: A retrospective study. *Criminal Justice and Behavior, 42*(11), 1183–1199. doi:10.1177/0093854815595662

Miller, K. M. (2006). The impact of parental incarceration on children: An emerging need for effective interventions. *Child and Adolescent Social Work Journal, 23*(4), 472–486. doi:10.1007/s10560-006-0065-6

Minnesota Department of Education. (2015). *Minnesota Student Survey.* Retrieved from http://education.state.mn.us/MDE/StuSuc/SafeSch/MNStudentSurvey/

Murphey, D., & Cooper, P. M. (2015). *Parents behind bars*. Retrieved from http://www.childtrends.org/wp-content/uploads/2015/10/2015-42ParentsBehindBars.pdf

Murray, J., & Farrington, D. P. (2005). Parental imprisonment: Effects on boys' antisocial behaviour and delinquency through the life-course. *Journal of Child Psychology and Psychiatry, 46*(12), 1269–1278. doi:10.1111/j.1469-7610.2005.01433.x

Murray, J., & Farrington, D. P. (2008). The effects of parental imprisonment on children. In M. Tonry (Ed.), *Crime and justice: A review of research* (pp. 133–206). Chicago, IL: University of Chicago Press.

Murray, J., Janson, C.-G., & Farrington, D. P. (2007). Crime in adult offspring of prisoners: A cross-national comparison of two longitudinal samples. *Criminal Justice and Behavior, 34*(1), 133–149. doi:10.1177/0093854806289549

Murray, J., Loeber, R., & Pardini, D. (2012). Parental involvement in the criminal justice system and the development of youth theft, marijuana use, depression, and poor academic performance. *Criminology, 50*(1), 255–302. doi:10.1111/j.1745-9125.2011.00257.x

Poehlmann, J., & Eddy, J. M. (2010). A research and intervention agenda for children of incarcerated parents. In J. M. Eddy, & J. Poehlmann (Eds.), *Children of incarcerated parents: A handbook for researchers and practitioners* (pp. 237–261). Washington, DC: Urban Institute Press.

Rodriguez, N. (2013). Concentrated disadvantage and the incarceration of youth: Examining how context affects juvenile justice. *Journal of Research in Crime and Delinquency, 50*(2), 189–215. doi:10.1177/0022427811425538

Shlafer, R. J., & Poehlmann, J. (2010). Children of incarcerated parents: Attachment relationships and behavioral outcomes. *Attachment & Human Development, 12*(4), 395–415. doi:10.1080/14616730903417052

Slade, E. P., Stuart, E. A., Salkever, D. S., Karakus, M., Green, K. M., & Ialongo, N. (2008). Impacts of age of onset of substance use disorders on risk of adult incarceration among disadvantaged urban youth: A propensity score matching approach. *Drug and Alcohol Dependence, 95*, 1–13. doi:10.1016/j.drugalcdep.2007.11.019

Stoolmiller, M., & Blechman, E. A. (2005). Substance use is a robust predictor of adolescent recidivism. *Criminal Justice and Behavior, 32*(3), 302–328. doi:10.1177/0093854804274372

Teplin, L. A., Abram, K. M., McClelland, G. M., Dulcan, M. K., & Mericle, A. A. (2002). Psychiatric disorders in youth in juvenile detention. *Archives of General Psychiatry, 59*(12), 1133–1143. doi:10.1001/archpsyc.60.11.1097

Travis, J., McBride, E. C., & Solomon, A. L. (2005). *Families left behind: The hidden costs of incarceration and reentry*. Retrieved from http://www.urban.org/Template.cfm?Section=ByAuthor&NavMenuID=63&template=/TaggedContent/ViewPublication.cfm&PublicationID=8633

Turney, K., & Haskins, A. R. (2014). Falling behind? Children's early grade retention after paternal incarceration. *Sociology of Education, 87*(4), 241–258. doi:10.1177/0038040714547086

University of Washington Social Development Research Group. (n.d.). *Families Facing the Future*. Retrieved from http://www.sdrg.org/fffsummary.asp

Wakefield, S., & Uggen, C. (2010). Incarceration and stratification. *Annual Review of Sociology, 36*(1), 387–406. doi:10.1146/annurev.soc.012809.102551

Williams, R. J., & Nowatzki, N. (2005). Validity of adolescent self-report of substance use. *Substance Use & Misuse, 40*(3), 299–311. doi:10.1081/JA-200049327

Zhang, Y., Maxwell, C. D., & Vaughn, M. S. (2009). The impact of state sentencing policies on the U.S. prison population. *Journal of Criminal Justice, 37*(2), 190–199. doi:10.1016/j.jcrimjus.2009.02.012

Variations in the Life Histories of Incarcerated Parents by Race and Ethnicity: Implications for Service Provision

Keva M. Miller, PhD, J. Mark Eddy, PhD, Sharon Borja, MSW, and Sarah R. Lazzari, MS

ABSTRACT

Incarcerated parents have complex life histories that often remain unresolved during incarceration, can continue to create barriers to prosocial success on release, and present similar intergenerational challenges for their children. This study examines the life histories of incarcerated fathers and mothers from the Pacific Northwest and how their experiences vary based on race and ethnicity. Five areas examined were exposure to trauma, child welfare involvement, mental health and substance abuse problems, juvenile justice and adult criminal justice involvement, and intergenerational criminal justice involvement. The sample comprised 359 incarcerated parents, and their racial/ethnic composition was 59% White, 14% African American, 11% multiracial, 8% Native American, and 7% Latino. Few differences were found across racial and ethnic groups. Mothers appeared more similar to each other across groups than fathers. Results illustrated similarities yet some surprising differences with national trends on key study variables. Implications for future research and intervention and prevention are discussed.

Concern for public safety, the deleterious effects of crime on communities, and overall discontentment with criminal justice, including penal policies, are highly publicized national issues. During the past four decades, ideologies about crime and sanctions against people who commit crime shifted from a rehabilitative focus to one of punishment (Gartner & Kruttschnitt, 2004). As a result, the United States today has the highest incarceration rate in the world, with nearly 2.2 million incarcerated people in local and county jails and state or federal prisons (Carson & Sabol, 2012; The Sentencing Project, 2013; The Pew Center on the States, 2008), the majority of whom are parents to children they resided with before their arrests, have direct contact with their children during the incarceration period, and will likely return to their parenting roles once released (Maruschak, Glaze, & Mumola, 2010; Eddy & Poehlmann, 2010).

Many incarcerated parents have life histories that include violence and ongoing abuse, exploitation, enduring trauma, mental health issues, and substance abuse problems—all of which increase their risk for the commission of additional crimes after release and increase their children's risk of immediate- and long-term problems (DeHart, 2008; Miller, 2014; Miller & Bank, 2013; Miller, Orellana, Johnson, Krase, & Anderson-Nathe, 2013). For incarcerated parents of color, exposure to these vulnerabilities is greater as it is well documented that people of color are disproportionately more likely to live in economically disadvantaged communities affected by significantly more adverse conditions. Unfortunately, the evidence base on the effectiveness of interventions that might help mitigate the impact of adverse conditions for incarcerated parents and their children is severely limited (Murray, Farrington, & Sekol, 2012; Murray, Loeber, & Pardini, 2012). The most common area of intervention focus has been on parenting. However, even for this topic there are a few evaluations of outcomes that use experimental designs (see Eddy & Poehlmann, 2010). A prominent gap in the literature is any rigorous evaluation of the appropriateness of the interventions that have been studied for various racial, ethnic and cultural groups in the United States. Unfortunately, the research base that might help inform intervention development for such groups is also limited. Few examinations have been conducted on the life experiences that potentially place specific racial, ethnic, and cultural groups at greater risks for continued struggles post-release.

This article provides an overview of the characteristics of incarcerated fathers and mothers and their life experiences by race and ethnicity. Examining similarities and differences based on race and ethnicity provides crucial information to consider in the development of culturally responsive and effective interventions. Of particular interest to us is information that will inform the creation of a tailored approach that best fits the needs of a particular family and that addresses not only the prerelease and postrelease needs of parents and their families but also strengthens parent–child relationships and ultimately reduces the risk of recidivism.

Background

In recent years, discussions concerning burgeoning incarceration rates have led to concerted efforts to better understand pathways to incarceration and to identify intervention strategies that divert progress along such pathways, assist transformative behaviors during incarceration, and provide skills and knowledge that contribute to successful reentry. Unfortunately, too few prison-based programs exist that adequately address the complexities of the challenges that were present before incarceration. Thus, numerous issues in the lives of offenders often remain unresolved during incarceration, and significant vulnerabilities remain on release that are likely to create barriers to prosocial success after release. Here, we review what is known about some of these vulnerabilities.

Childhood exposure to trauma and child welfare involvement

Trauma histories from childhood are prevalent among incarcerated populations. For example, in a study of incarcerated individuals with drug dependence, women reported greater exposure to childhood trauma, with 40% of women reporting emotional abuse and neglect, 29% reporting physical abuse, and 39% experiencing sexual abuse compared with 20%, 20%, and 9% of men, respectively (Messina, Grella, Burdon, & Prendergast, 2007). In separate studies, more than 60% of women reported having experienced childhood trauma (Green, Miranda, Daroowalla, & Siddique, 2005), while almost 45% of men in state prison reported physical trauma, with Whites reporting higher prevalence than African Americans, Latinos, and American Indians (Wolff & Shi, 2012).

The high rates of childhood victimization reported in multiple studies serve as evidence of a common experience of a trauma, including exposures to multiple types of victimization. Such experiences may have led to child welfare system involvement, physical removal from their families, and subsequent experiences with numerous ephemeral foster care placements (Messina et al., 2007). Nationally, children of color in particular are disproportionately overrepresented in the child welfare system compared with their representation in the general population, and disparately represented in the system compared with White children (Sedlak & Broadhurst, 1996; Sedlak et al., 2010; Sedlak & Schultz, 2005; U.S. General Accounting Office, 2007). Additionally, data show that African American children are overrepresented in child welfare systems in all 50 states, American Indian children in 24 states, and Latino children in 10 states (Hill, Jackson, & Waheed, 2008). It is unclear whether there is a connection between the overrepresentation of children of color in the child welfare system and the overrepresentation of incarcerated parents of color, as few studies have examined potential links between these phenomena (Miller & Bank, 2013).

Adult exposure to trauma

Studies have shown that people with criminal justice involvement have high rates of lifetime exposure for any type of violence, ranging between 43% and 92% among men and between 60% and 99% among women (Breslau, 2009; Cook, Smith, Tusher, & Raiford, 2005; Reichert, Adams, & Bostwick, 2010).

Among adults, partner violence is among the most common form of victimization, with an average as high as 90% of incarcerated women having experienced physical or sexual partner violence (Green et al., 2005; Lynch, Fritch, & Heath, 2012). In a later study involving incarcerated parents, almost half of male inmates and more than 70% of female inmates reported experiences of physical violence, while at least 33% reported sexual abuse by a family member (Carlson & Shafer, 2010). High rates of victimization in childhood and adulthood point to a potentially greater prevalence of polyvictimization among institutionalized populations compared with the general population. The previously mentioned studies also highlight women as having experienced a greater degree of victimization than men, with potentially more substantial life histories of multiple victimization.

While some studies have tested the hypothesized links between earlier victimization to later revictimization, much more is to be learned from the prison population about the extent to which later revictimization impacts their lives. Scholars have pointed to the high risk for retraumatization by events related to the process of corrections involvement and from acute and chronic situations that can occur while residing within the prison environment (Bloom, Owen, & Covington, 2004). Unfortunately, very little information is available on any of these topics for minority incarcerated men or women.

Mental health and substance abuse problems

Ongoing mental health and substance abuse problems are often directly associated with enduring trauma that begins during childhood and extends into adulthood. The risks for ongoing mental health and substance abuse issues can be exacerbated by the trauma associated with facing years of incarceration, coping with the physical and emotional separation from family and friends, and adapting to prison life. Many men and women in correctional facilities who report lifelong traumatic experiences are often diagnosed with or report mental health and/or substance abuse problems. Research suggests that incarcerated individuals are disproportionately affected by mental health and substance abuse problems compared with the general population (Fazel, Bains, & Doll, 2006; Fazel & Danesh, 2002; Hammett, Roberts, & Kennedy, 2001).

A national level study found that of the incarcerated parents confined in state facilities, 57% had mental health problems and 67% had substance abuse or dependence problems (Glaze & Maruschak, 2008). Analyses of the racial or ethnic makeup of mental health and substance abuse prevalence rates among the sample were not performed. In another national study of incarcerated adults, mental health concerns were more common among Whites, with 62% of state and 71% of jailed White inmates meeting criteria for mental illness (James & Glaze, 2006). Individuals categorized as "other" (identified as either American Indian, Alaskan Native, Pacific Islander, or mixed race) had the second highest percentages, with 62% of state and 70% of jailed racially identified "other" inmates had mental health concerns. Incarcerated Hispanics in all settings were the least likely to have a mental health concern.

Juvenile justice involvement

Exposure to trauma and related mental health and substance abuse problems are some of the most common predictors for criminal activity and subsequent involvement in the justice system, including during youth. Most research in juvenile justice on the association between trauma experiences and justice involvement has focused on girls (Chesney-Lind, Morash, & Stevens, 2008; Gavazzi, Yarcheck, & Chesney-Lind, 2006). Delinquency among girls, in particular, is often hypothesized to be one outcome of exposure to trauma (Cauffman, 2008; Pasko & Mayeda, 2011; Seigel & Williams, 2003). Girls who come to the attention of the juvenile justice system are affected by prior emotional neglect, physical abuse, and sexual abuse/violence or sexual exploitation at higher rates than their peers (Schaffner, 2007; Widom, 2000). Further, many of these girls may have been exposed to parental substance abuse/dependence, parental criminality and criminal justice involvement, and/or multiple temporary foster care placements (Acoca, 1998; Belknap & Holsinger, 2006).

The issues associated with racial disparity in the juvenile justice system are mutlifaceted and not easily deconstructed by attributing them to a single factor (Miller, Anderson-Nathe, & Meinhold, 2014). Regardless of the contributors of systems involvement, youth of color, in particular African American boys and girls, are disproportionately represented at all stages of system engagement—from arrest all the way to secure confinement (Armstrong & Rodriguez, 2005; Bishop, 2005; Crutchfield, Skinner, Haggerty, McGlynn, & Catalano, 2009; Puzzanchera & Adams, 2012; Shook & Goodkind, 2009). Compared with White youth, African American youth have the most evident disparity, such that African American youth were 123% more likely to be arrested, 43% more likely to be detained, and 23% more likely to be placed in secure facilities (Puzzanchera & Adams, 2012).

Intergenerational incarceration

Historically, research has focused on understanding the link between parent criminality and the long-term, intergenerational impact on children (see, for example, Gottfredson & Hirschi, 1990; Murray & Farrignton, 2005; Roettger & Swisher, 2009). More recent literature has begun to focus on parental incarceration, such as the number of times a parent has been incarcerated (Miller & Bank, 2013) and how the dynamic of multiple encounters of family members with the correctional system affects intergenerational criminality (Perry & Bright, 2012; Roettger & Swisher, 2009; Wildeman & Western, 2010). Glaze and Maruschak (2008) found that 49% of men and 58% of women in state prisons had a close relative with a history of incarceration. For communities of color, intergenerational incarceration is of particular concern (Wildeman & Western, 2010). Clear (2007) refers to an increasing number of impoverished communities with high minority populations as "prison places" where young people of color, and in particular African American and Latino men, are significantly more likely to spend time behind bars than are their White counterparts (Clear, 2007; Roettger & Swisher, 2009; Wildeman & Western, 2010).

Purpose of the study

This study is intended to build on the literature reviewed and explores the life histories of parents incarcerated within a state prison system and how their experiences vary based on race and ethnicity. Five areas are examined: child welfare experiences, trauma exposure, mental health and substance abuse problems, juvenile justice and adult criminal justice involvement, and intergenerational criminal justice involvement.

Method

Study overview

Data came from the initial assessment of the Parent Child Study, a randomized controlled trial of Parenting Inside Out (PIO), a research-informed cognitive-behavioral parent management training program developed for incarcerated mothers and fathers (Eddy et al., 2008; Eddy, Martinez, & Burraston, 2013). The study was conducted within four facilities (three for men, one for women, and the only one in the state) operated by the Oregon Department of Corrections (DOC), all of which operated at minimum or medium levels of security. Participants had to be parents who had past and current social connection to their children (see later). Women and racial and/or ethnic minority inmates were oversampled from an eligible pool of participants to increase the representation of these groups, with a goal of 50% female and 50% racial/ethnic minority participants in the sample. Participants were individually randomized, blocking on gender and on race/ethnicity, into a PIO "intervention" condition or a services as usual "control" condition, and were assessed multiple times during and after release from prison. The study was conducted with the approval and oversight of the federal Office of Human Research Protections and the nonprofit Oregon Social Learning Center (OSLC) Institutional Review Board.

Participants

The sample comprises 359 participants who were recruited from all DOC facilities throughout the state. About half of participants were women (54%) and were White (59%). The minority racial and ethnic groups in the sample included 14% African American, 11% multiracial, 8% Native American, and 7% Hispanic White (hereafter referred to as Latino). Approximately 60% of participants had less than a high school education, 13% had a high school diploma or GED, and the remainder had at least some additional training or education after high school. The typical parent had three children, most of whom were biological children. The average child was 8 years old. In the month before their current incarceration, 35% of parents had lived with their children full-time and 9% part-time, 18% visited with their children at least once a week, 14% had visited less than once a week, and the rest had little or no contact. These percentages were similar for men and women. Men were more likely to have been sentenced for a person crime (61% versus 40%), to be serving longer sentences than women (2.2 years versus 1.5 years), and to have been in the custody of the DOC a greater number of times (1.7 versus 1.4). In contrast, women were more likely to have been older than men the first time they were arrested as an adult (23 years versus 20 years). Most participants had histories of drug and/or alcohol abuse or addiction (87% of men and 93% of women), and many had histories of other mental health problems (27% of men and 45% of women). Almost 55% of participants had a parent and 53% had a sibling who had spent some time in jail or prison. Most also had a parent (70%) or a sibling (61%) who had had problems with drugs or alcohol at some point during their lives.

Eligibility

To be eligible for participation in the study, an inmate was required to have (a) at least one child between the ages of 3 and 11 years, (b) the legal right to contact their child, (c) had some role in parenting their children in the past and expected some such role in the future, (d) not committed either a crime against a child or any type of sex offense, (e) contact information for the caregiver of at least one of his/her young children, and (f) less than 9 months remaining before the end of their prison sentence.

Recruitment

During a 3-year recruitment period, potential participants within each of the 14 correctional units within the Oregon DOC were informed about the study through a variety of means, including postings in correctional institution newspapers, signs on bulletin boards, announcements during inmate club meetings, and special meetings about the study. Inmates were invited to send a letter through prison mail to the research team if they were interested in the study. Of the 1483 inmates who expressed interest in the study and were screened, 453 were eligible. The most common reasons for ineligibility were no children in the appropriate age range and release dates that were too distant. Approximately 80% of eligible inmates consented to participate in the study. If these individuals did not live in a study institution, a request was made to transfer them; most transfers were granted. There was a significant difference in participation by sex, with 68% of eligible men and 92% of eligible women participating. The majority of men (66%) who chose not to participate did so because they did not want to transfer away from their current institution. Men who were not residing in one of the three participating institutions for men were transferred there after they were enrolled in the study.

Measures

At the initial assessment before the start of the intervention, participants in the control and intervention conditions were interviewed across two occasions on their background experiences before and during prison, with a particular focus on their family relationships. Parents received $30 for their participation in this assessment. Each of the dependent variables of interest in this report were measured with single-item questions that have been commonly asked in past surveys of incarcerated parents and had face validity. The independent variable, race/ethnicity, was coded based on self-identification as (non-Hispanic) White, (non-Hispanic) African American, Latino (all Hispanic White), Native American, or other (i.e., 85% multiracial, 12% other race/ethnicity, and 3% Asian/Pacific Islander).

Analytic strategy

Chi-square tests were computed for men and for women with race/ethnicity as the independent variable and various life history situations coded in categories as dependent variables. Analyses of variance (ANOVAs) were computed comparing means on continuous variables, and post-hoc tests were conducted if appropriate.

Results

Few of the tests conducted were significant, suggesting that, within sex, the members of the racial and ethnic groups examined were relatively similar to each other in terms of the aspects of life history described by the variables used here (see Table 1). Across the groups, women appeared to be more

Table 1. Incarcerated Parent Life Histories by Race/Ethnicity.

		White %, x̄ (SD)	African American %, x̄ (SD)	American Indian %, x̄ (SD)	Latino %, x̄ (SD)	Others %, x̄ (SD)	Total %, x̄ (SD)	p
N		214	46	28	28	43	359	
Mental health and substance abuse problems								
Ever experienced mental health	Men	29.7	24.0	46.2	20.0	10.5	27.2	0.223
	Women	49.6	23.8	40.0	33.3	54.2	45.2	0.149
Ever diagnosed with a mental health problems	Men	51.1ᵃ⁺	32.0	53.8	10.0ᵃ⁻	31.6	43.4	0.045*
	Women	54.2	14.3ᵃ⁻	46.7	55.6	75.0ᵃ⁺	52.0	0.002**
Ever experienced drug and/or alcohol abuse or addiction	Men	93.4ᵃ⁺	76.0	84.6	90.0	68.4	86.7	0.020*
	Women	95.0	81.0	92.9	100.00	91.7	93.4	0.130
Trauma/victimization								
Hit by a partner	Men	64.8	52.0	76.9	30.0	63.2	61.4	0.142
	Women	77.3	76.2	66.7	83.3	79.2	77.2	0.845
Physically hurt by a romantic partner	Men	34.1	24.0	30.8	30.0	26.3	31.0	0.883
	Women	70.6	66.7	66.7	77.8	75.0	71.1	0.921
Sexually assaulted	Men	15.4	4.0	23.1	0.0	11.1	12.8	0.301
	Women	48.6	36.8	61.5	64.7	60.9	51.4	0.341
Child welfare involvement								
Foster care	Men	26.1	16.0	15.4	0.0	26.3	22.0	0.346
	Women	26.5	28.6	40.0	22.2	29.2	27.7	0.823
Group home	Men	27.2	32.0	7.7	0.0	26.3	24.7	0.197
	Women	18.8	38.1	28.6	11.1	17.4	20.7	0.214
Residential treatment	Men	30.8ᵃ⁺	4.0ᵃ⁻	25.0	15.4	11.1	22.6	0.037*
	Women	28.2	10.5	21.4	12.5	13.0	22.5	0.223
Juvenile justice history								
Arrested as a child or adolescent	Men	75.0	84.0	46.2	20.0ᵃ⁻	68.4	69.8	0.001**
	Women	46.2	57.1	50.0	41.2	41.7	46.7	0.836
Times arrested	Men	12.40 (16.70)	6.38 (7.81)	4.50 (7.60)	1.50 (0.70)	5.33 (8.67)	9.80 (14.34)	0.195
	Women	6.59 (9.20)	8.58 (14.0)	10.83 (19.28)	11.16 (11.23)	10.70 (11.66)	7.93 (11.09)	0.677
Spent time in lock-up	Men	59.8	72.0	15.4	11.1ᵃ⁻	63.2	55.7	0.001**
	Women	29.9	42.9	33.3	16.7	33.3	30.8	0.512

(Continued)

Table 1. (Continued).

		White		African American		American Indian		Latino		Others		Total		p
		%, x̄	(SD)	%, x̄	(SD)	%, x̄	(SD)	%, x̄	(SD)	%, x̄	(SD)	%, x̄	(SD)	
Times in lock-up	Men	7.92	(13.55)	3.11	(2.78)	1.00	(0.00)	1.00	(.)	3.25	(6.56)	6.02	(6.56)	0.402
	Women	4.36	(4.88)	5.88	(8.08)	17.66	(28.0)	7.66	(4.04)	10.50	(10.59)	6.27	(8.72)	0.060
Adult criminal history														
Times arrested	Men	21.18	(30.20)	25.29	(39.69)	10.23	(10.14)	13.20	(13.71)	20.21	(21.51)	20.27	(29.09)	0.573
	Women	12.75	(15.37)	15.25	(23.59)	11.13	(15.34)	10.83	(11.16)	19.09	(21.25)	13.43	(16.80)	0.462
Average times locked-up	Men	14.33	(18.84)	17.09	(14.29)	8.91	(11.39)	6.11	(3.62)	17.56	(23.08)	14.24	(17.77)	0.398
	Women	8.70	(9.96)	14.63	(21.88)	9.85	(15.94)	7.64	(10.33)	13.88	(18.13)	9.82	(13.14)	0.314
Intergenerational incarceration														
Parental incarceration	Men	55.6		63.6		57.1		25.0		40.0		53.2		0.626
	Women	59.3		54.5		75.0		66.7		62.5		60.5		0.951
Grandparental incarceration	Men	23.3		32.0		25.0		10.0		11.1		22.6		0.463
	Women	23.1		19.0		14.3		17.6		18.2		20.9		0.917
Three generations of incarceration	Men	5.2		10.0		18.2		10.0		0.0		6.7		0.359
	Women	8.7		5.6		0.0		11.8		14.3		8.7		0.665

Note. * = p<.05. ** = p<.01. a± = Adjusted standardized residual ±2.

similar to each other than men (only 1 of 19 tests significant versus 5 of 19, respectively). For women, the one significant test was for the relation between race/ethnicity and ever diagnosed with a mental health problem, with this value being greater than the average (i.e., adjusted standardized residual for the cell greater than +2.0) for those in the "other race/ethnicity" group and less than average (i.e., adjusted standardized residual for the cell less than −2.0) for African Americans. For men, this test was also significant, with Whites greater than average and Latinos less than average. Further, for men, race/ethnicity was also related to ever experienced drug and alcohol addiction (with Whites, again, higher than the average based on the adjusted standardized residuals), spent time in residential treatment during adolescence (Whites higher, African Americans lower), and as a juvenile, detained by police and spent time in lock-up (less than average for Latinos).

For men, beyond the significant findings, there was a pattern of findings that seemed to stand out. Looking at the groups that had the very highest and lowest scores (i.e., percentages or means) for the variables considered, White men had problems in a variety of areas. In contrast, African American men were most notable for their involvement in the justice system, as juveniles and adults. American Indian men were most notable for their high scores in the area of mental health problems and trauma. Latinos had the lowest scores on most every variable except for drug and alcohol addiction. The "other" group were also low on almost every variable examined except for involvement in child welfare/foster care. These patterns were subtle, however, as variation on many of the variables across race and ethnicity was not wide, and again, few significant differences were observed. For women, as might be expected from the lack of significant findings, the picture was less clear, with each group having some of the highest and some of the lowest values for several variables.

Discussion

The current study builds on the existing knowledge base regarding complex and challenging circumstances that are known to negatively affect the lives of incarcerated men and women and increase their children's risk for potentially devastating outcomes. Here, the focus was specifically on parents and whether there were reliable differences between parents of different racial and ethnic groups. In this Pacific Northwest sample, many similarities were found in the life histories of incarcerated parents across groups, especially among incarcerated mothers.

The study findings replicate a variety of prior findings. For example, high rates of involvement with the child welfare and juvenile justice systems are well documented among African American incarcerated fathers and African American and American Indian incarcerated mothers, and such was found here. This multisystem involvement, combined with the observed intergenerational pattern of incarceration and the short- and long-term consequences of such among these subpopulations, point to the high risks that the children of these particular incarcerated parents face.

Consistent with other studies, White men reported higher rates of adult physical abuse/trauma and mental health and substance abuse problems compared with African American, Latino, and "other" men. Notably, however, American Indian fathers and Latino mothers were the most likely to report histories of abuse by a domestic partner and/or sexual assault. This set of problems place the children of these incarcerated parents vulnerable to a different set of problems that may lead to similar outcomes. Ultimately, the incarcerated parents in this sample may be the victims and the architects (cf. Patterson, 1976) of situations that for themselves and for their children lead to both becoming involved in systems that are intended to remediate problems but unfortunately are not particularly effective at doing so—whether that be the child welfare system, the juvenile justice system, or the criminal justice system.

The narrative that seems to emerge from these findings is that incarcerated parents' prior histories may vary to some degree by race and ethnicity but only to the extent that they are related to issues that are experienced widely within their identified racial or ethnic group. In the case of African Americans in this sample, for example, this unfortunately means a greater likelihood of ongoing justice system involvement and the short- and long-term consequences of such. In the case of American Indians, this may mean longer histories of trauma and abuse, including traumas that were not assessed, such as intergenerational historical trauma.

While the majority of life history indicators showed similar trends as in past studies, there were a few unexpected findings related to race and ethnicity that merit attention. In contrast to national child welfare statistics as well as regional child welfare statistics from the area in which this study sample was recruited (e.g., Miller, Cahn, & Orellana, 2012; Sedlak et al., 2010), relatively high rates of child welfare involvement were found among White incarcerated men and women and relatively high rates of juvenile justice involvement among White incarcerated men. These differences may be due to how the sample was recruited (e.g., parents with specific types of involvement with their children), random variation, or some other reason. Unfortunately, few studies of incarcerated parents per se are available with which to compare.

Implications for practice and research

The relative lack of differences between racial and ethnic groups on the various life history experiences assessed here does not mean that there are not important issues that should be considered when developing and delivering preventive and intervention services for the children of incarcerated parents and their families. Rather, this finding points to the relatively limited number of pathways that lead to criminal justice involvement. There are a fewer number of ways to get in trouble in the United States and end up incarcerated than there are ways to succeed and end up living a successful life in the community. Variation is much greater on the positive side of life than on the negative.

This particular investigation focused on elements that are common components of a pathway to crime and punishment, including trauma, mental health problems, substance use and abuse, and failure at multiple points that leads to system involvement and the consequences of such, including isolation from prosocial opportunities. Historical elements that were not examined here, such as involvement in specific cultural practices and other potential strengths, might paint a different picture on how the members of these various racial and ethnic groups differ from each other.

A key issue that may be magnified in a sample this small is that the variation within each of these groups is likely to be much greater than the variation within the groups. Clustering individuals into a category, like "Latino," creates a convenient classification for a study like this but hides the fact that such a term encompasses a tremendously varied group of peoples who differ in many important ways from each other but in the United States are considered one "group." A more adequate consideration of how race and ethnicity might be important in prevention and intervention would need to include thinking more deeply about a variety of other issues, including but not limited to community, region and country of origin, time in the United States, and religious beliefs, and to do this would require a much larger sample that was recruited from a variety of urban and rural sites around the country.

While this study found few clear differences between White incarcerated parents and incarcerated parents of color, given the overrepresentation of people of color in child welfare and juvenile justice systems in particular, future research must continue to examine how race poses increased risks for a lifelong entrenchment in systems of care and confinement. Special attention must be given to how these risks transfer to the children of incarcerated parents of color. Further research is needed on services and interventions that focus on multiple points in the life course when individuals come to the attention of systems, including early trauma and child welfare involvement, early antisocial behavior and school and juvenile justice system involvement, and later antisocial behavior and criminal justice involvement. However, taking this type of reactive approach, after a problem has come to the attention of authorities, has not and will not be sufficient for adequately addressing the needs in our society. Based on a limited but accruing database, complementary primary and secondary prevention approaches have great potential to reduce the numbers of children and families in need of more resource intensive interventions, and creative, diligent, and persistent research efforts are needed on examining when and how these can make a difference in the lives of children affected by incarceration, including children of color.

Limitations

While the sample used here was much more racially and ethnically diverse than the Oregon state prison population, the proportional representation of racial and ethnic groups in this study is not reflective of that of incarcerated parents nationally. Further, participants were asked to retrospectively provide life history accounts, which may have affected the accuracy of various aspects of their reports, including their occurrence and temporal relations.

Conclusion

A significant proportion of incarcerated fathers and mothers from all races and ethnicities experience some combination of difficult life history experiences, whether that be trauma, victimization, juvenile justice involvement, diagnosed and/or undiagnosed mental health problems, substance abuse issues, and/or intergenerational incarceration. These findings support the critical need, for men and women of all racial and ethnic groups, for preventive interventions for men and women that divert individuals from pathways that lead to crime and criminal justice involvement and assist in skill and life history building that lead to prosocial outcomes. To be effective, such interventions need to address the factors that affect a particular man or woman, including those factors that may be related to race and ethnicity. Once incarcerated, the findings highlight the need for considering life histories and their implications for future success and addressing these in an appropriate and effective manner while simultaneously helping overcome traditional barriers faced during reentry (e.g., lack of housing, employment, prosocial support).

Acknowledgments

Special appreciation and gratitude are extended to the incarcerated parents and their families for their participation in this study.

Funding

The work was supported by grants MH46690 and MH6553 from the Division of Epidemiology and Services Research, National Institute of Mental Health, National Institutes of Health (NIH), U.S. Public Health Service (PHS); by grant HD054480 from the Social and Affective Development/Child Maltreatment and Violence, National Institute of Child Health and Human Development, NIH, U.S. PHS; by a grant from the Edna McConnell Clark Foundation; and by funding from the legislature of the state of Oregon.

References

Acoca, L. (1998). Outside/inside: The violation of American girls at home, in the streets, and in the system. *Crime and Delinquency*, *44*(4), 561–590. doi:10.1177/0011128798044004006

Armstrong, G. S., & Rodriguez, N. (2005). Effects of individual and contextual characteristics on preadjudication detention of juvenile delinquents. *Justice Quarterly*, *22*(4), 521–539. doi:10.1080/07418820500364643

Belknap, J., & Holsinger, K. (2006). The gendered nature of risk factors for delinquency. *Feminist Criminology*, *1*(1), 48–71. doi:10.1177/1557085105282897

Bishop, D. M. (2005). The role of race and ethnicity in juvenile justice processing. In D. F. Hawkins, & K. Kempf-Leonard (Eds.), *Our children, their children* (pp. 23–82). Chicago, IL: University of Chicago Press.

Breslau, N. (2009). The epidemiology of trauma, PTSD, and other posttrauma disorders. *Trauma Violence Abuse*, *10*, 198–210. doi:10.1177/1524838009334448

Carlson, B. E., & Shafer, M. S. (2010). Traumatic histories and stressful life events of incarcerated parents: Childhood and adult trauma histories. *The Prison Journal*, *90*(4), 494–515. doi:10.1177/0032885510382226

Carson, E. A. & Sabol, W. J. (2012). *Prisoners in 2011*. Washington: DC: Office of Justice Programs, Bureau of Justice Statistics, U.S. Department of Justice.

Cauffman, E. (2008). Understanding the female offender. *The Future of Children*, *18*(2), 119–142. doi:10.1353/foc.0.0015

Chesney-Lind, M., Morash, M., & Stevens, T. (2008). Girls troubles, girls' delinquency, and gender responsive programming: A review. *Australian & New Zealand Journal of Criminology*, *41*(1), 162–189. doi:10.1375/acri.41.1.162

Clear, T. R. (2007). *Imprisoning communities: How mass incarceration makes disadvantaged neighborhoods worse*. New York, NY: Oxford University Press.

Cook, S. L., Smith, S. G., Tusher, C. P., & Raiford, J. (2005). Self-reports of traumatic events in a random sample of incarcerated women. *Women & Criminal Justice*, *16*(1/2), 107–125. doi:10.1300/J012v16n01_05

Crutchfield, R. D., Skinner, M. L., Haggerty, K. P., McGlynn, A., & Catalano, R. F. (2009). Racial disparities in early criminal justice involvement. *Race and Social Problems*, *1*(4), 218–230. doi:10.1007/s12552-009-9018-y

DeHart, D. D. (2008). Pathways to prison: Impact of victimization in the lives of incarcerated women. *Violence Against Women*, *14*, 1362–1381. doi:10.1177/1077801208327018

Eddy, J. M., Martinez, C. R., Jr., & Burraston, B. (2013). A randomized controlled trial of a parent management training program for incarcerated parents: Proximal impacts. *Monographs of the Society for Research in Child Development*, *78*(3), 75–93.

Eddy, J. M., Martinez, C. R., Jr., Schiffmann, T., Newton, R., Olin, L., & Shortt, J. (2008). Development of a multisystemic parent management training intervention for incarcerated parents, their children and families. *Clinical Psychologist, 12*(3), 86–98. doi:10.1080/13284200802495461

Eddy, J. M., & Poehlmann, J. (Eds.). (2010). *Children of incarcerated parents: A handbook for researchers and practitioners.* Washington, DC: Urban Institute Press.

Fazel, S., Bains, P., & Doll, H. (2006). Substance abuse and dependence in prisoners: A systematic review. *Addiction, 101*(2), 181–191. doi:10.1111/add.2006.101.issue-2

Fazel, S., & Danesh, J. (2002). Serious mental disorder in 23,000 prisoners: A systematic review of 62 surveys. *The Lancet, 359*(9306), 545–550. doi:10.1016/S0140-6736(02)07740-1

Gartner, R., & Kruttschnitt, C. (2004). A brief history of doing time: The California Institution for Women in the 1960s and the 1990s. *Law & Society Review, 38*(2), 267–304. doi:10.1111/j.0023-9216.2004.03802009.x

Gavazzi, S. M., Yarcheck, C. M., & Chesney-Lind, M. (2006). Global risk indicators and the role of gender in a juvenile detention sample. *Criminal Justice and Behavior, 33*(5), 597–612. doi:10.1177/0093854806288184

Glaze, L. E., & Maruschak, L. M. (2008). *Parents in prison and their minor children.* Washington, DC: U.S. Department of Justice.

Gottfredson, M. R., & Hirschi, T. (1990). *A general theory of crime.* Stanford, CA: Stanford University Press.

Green, B. L., Miranda, J., Daroowalla, A., & Siddique, J. (2005). Trauma exposure, mental health functioning, and program needs of women in jail. *Crime & Delinquency, 51*(1), 133–151. doi:10.1177/0011128704267477

Hammett, T. M., Roberts, C., & Kennedy, S. (2001). Health-related issues in prisoner reentry. *Crime & Delinquency, 47*(3), 390–409. doi:10.1177/0011128701047003006

Hill, R. B., Jackson, S., & Waheed, K. (2008, March). *Reducing racial and ethnic disproportionality and disparities in child welfare: Promoting racial equity.* Presentation at the Joint Meeting on Adolescent Treatment Effectiveness, Washington, DC.

James, D. J., & Glaze, L. E. (2006). *Mental health problems of prison and jail inmates* (Research Report No. 213600). Washington, DC: USDOJ.

Lynch, S. M., Fritch, A., & Heath, N. M. (2012). Looking beneath the surface the nature of incarcerated women's experiences of interpersonal violence, treatment needs, and mental health. *Feminist Criminology, 7*(4), 381–400. doi:10.1177/1557085112439224

Maruschak, L. M., Glaze, L. E., & Mumola, C. J. (2010). Incarcerated parents and their children: Findings from the bureau of justice statistics. In J. M. Eddy, & J. Poehlmann (Eds.), *Children of incarcerated parents: A handbook for researchers and practitioners* (pp. 33–54). Washington, DC: Urban Institute Press.

Messina, N., Grella, C., Burdon, W., & Prendergast, M. (2007). Childhood adverse events and current traumatic distress: A comparison of men and women drug-dependent prisoners. *Criminal Justice and Behavior, 34*(11), 1385–1401. doi:10.1177/0093854807305150

Miller, K. M. (2014). Maternal criminal justice involvement and co-occurring mental health and substance abuse problems: Examining moderation of sex and race on children's mental health. *Children and Youth Services Review, 37*, 71–80. doi:10.1016/j.childyouth.2013.12.008

Miller, K. M., Anderson-Nathe, B., & Meinhold, J. (2014). Gender and culturally grounded practice. In W. Church, D. W. Springer, & A. Roberts (Eds.), *Juvenile justice sourcebook: Past, present, and future* (2nd ed., pp. 581–606). New York, NY: Oxford University Press.

Miller, K. M., & Bank, L. (2013). Moderating effects of race on children's internalizing and externalizing behaviors who have mothers with child welfare and criminal justice involvement. *Children and Youth Services Review*, 35(3), 472–481. doi:10.1016/j.childyouth.2012.12.022

Miller, K. M., Cahn, K., & Orellana, E. R. (2012). Dynamics that contribute to racial disproportionality and disparity: Perspectives from child welfare professionals, community partners, and families. *Children and Youth Services Review*, 35(9), 2201–2207. doi:10.1016/j.childyouth.2012.07.022

Murray, J., & Farrington, D. P. (2005). Parental imprisonment: Effects on boys' antisocial behavior and delinquency through the life-course. *Journal of Child Psychology & Psychiatry*, 46, 1269–1278. doi:10.1111/j.1469-7610.2005.01433.x

Murray, J., Loeber, R., & Pardini, D. (2012). Parental involvement in the criminal justice system and the development of youth theft, depression, marijuana use, and poor academic performance. *Criminology*, 50(1), 255–302. doi:10.1111/j.1745-9125.2011.00257.x

Pasko, L., & Mayeda, D. T. (2011). Pathway and predictors of juvenile justice involvement for Native Hawaiian and Pacific Islander youth: A focus on gender. *Journal of Ethnic & Cultural Diversity in Social Work*, 20(2), 114–130. doi:10.1080/15313204.2011.570120

Patterson, G. R. (1976). The aggressive child: Victim and architect of a coercive system. In E. J. Mash, L. A. Hamerlynck, & L. C. Handy (Eds.), *Behavior modification and families: Theory and research* (Vol. 1, pp. 267–316). New York, NY: Brunner/Mazel.

Perry, A. R., & Bright, M. (2012). African American fathers and incarceration: Paternal involvement and child outcomes. *Social Work in Public Health*, 27, 187–203. doi:10.1080/19371918.2011.629856

The Pew Center. (2008). *One in 100: Behind bars in America*. Retrieved from www.pewcenteronthestatus.org/

Puzzanchera, C., & Adams, B. (2012). *National disproportionate minority contact databook*. Developed by the National Center for Juvenile Justice for the Office of Juvenile Justice and Delinquency Prevention. Retrieved from http://www.ojjdp.gov/ojstatbb/dmcdb/

Reichert, J., Adams, S., & Bostwick, L. (2010). *Victimization and help-seeking behaviors among women incarcerated in Illinois prisons* (pp. 1–75). Chicago, IL: Illinois Criminal Justice Reform Authority.

Roettger, M. E., & Swisher, R. R. (2009). *Examining racial variations in the associations of father's history of incarceration with son's delinquency and arrest in contemporary U.S. society* (Working Paper #09-01). Retrieved from http://ncfmr.bgsu.edu/pdf/Working%20Papers/wp09-01

Schaffner, L. (2007). Violence against girls provokes girls' violence: From private injury to public harm. *Violence Against Women*, 13(12), 1229–1248. doi:10.1177/1077801207309881

Sedlak, A., & Broadhurst, D. (1996). *Executive summary of the third National Incidence Study of Child Abuse and Neglect*. Washington, DC: U.S. Department of Health and Human Services.

Sedlak, A., & Schultz, D. (2005). Racial differences in child protective services investigation of abused and neglected children. In D. M. Derezotes, J. Poertner, & M. F. Testa (Eds.), *Race matters in child welfare: The overrepresentation of African American children in the system* (pp. 97–118). Washington, DC: Child Welfare League of America.

Sedlak, A. J., Mettenburg, J., Basena, M., Petta, I., McPherson, K., Greene, A., & Li, S. (2010). *Fourth national incidence study of child abuse and neglect (NIS–4): Report to Congress, executive summary*. Washington, DC: U. S. Department of Health and Human Services, Administration for Children and Families. Retrieved from http://www.acf.hhs.gov/programs/opre/abuse_neglect/natl_oncod/reports/natl_oncod/nis4_report_congress_full_pdf_jan2010.pdf

The Sentencing Project. (2013). *Report of the Sentencing Project to the United Nations Human Rights Committee: Regarding racial disparities in the United States criminal justice system*. Washington, DC: Author.

Shook, J. J., & Goodkind, S. (2009). Racial disproportionality in juvenile justice: The interaction of race and geography in pretrial detention for violent and serious offenses. *Race and Social Problems, 1*(4), 257–266. doi:10.1007/s12552-009-9021-3

Siegel, J. A., & Williams, L. M. (2003). The relationship between child sexual abuse and female delinquency and crime: A prospective study. *Journal of Research in Crime and Delinquency, 40*(1), 71–94. doi:10.1177/0022427802239254

U.S. General Accounting Office. (2007). *African American children in foster care: Additional HHS assistance needed to help states reduce the proportion in care* (GOA Publication No. GAO-07-816). Washington, DC: Author.

Widom, C. S. (2000). Childhood victimization: Early adversity, later psychopathology. *National Institute of Juvenile Justice Journal, 242*(1), 3–9.

Wildeman, C., & Western, B. (2010). Incarceration in fragile families. *Future of Children, 20*, 157–177. doi:10.1353/foc.2010.0006

Wolff, N., & Shi, J. (2012). Childhood and adult trauma experiences of incarcerated persons and their relationship to adult behavioral health problems and treatment. *International Journal of Environmental Research and Public Health, 9*(5), 1908–1926. doi:10.3390/ijerph9051908

A Statewide Parenting Alternative Sentencing Program: Description and Preliminary Outcomes

Chyla M. Aguiar, MA, and Susan Leavell

ABSTRACT
The Washington State Legislature created the Parenting Sentencing Alternative in 2010, authorizing a substitute to total confinement for parents of minor children. The Alternative is designed to strengthen family bonds and improve parenting skills to encourage successful reintegration. An overview of the Alternative's history, design, and implementation is presented, followed by preliminary results from an impact evaluation. A case study of a successful participant is presented, and implications for the findings are discussed.

The ethical, social, and fiscal problems created by the practice of mass incarceration during the past 40 years of American criminal justice policies are well established. Criminologists generally declare this practice to be *unsustainable* due to ever expanding operational costs (Clear & Frost, 2014; Currie, 2013), *unethical* because of the impact on disadvantaged communities and people of color (Clear, 2007; Reiman & Leighton, 2010; Walker, Spohn, & DeLone, 2012), and *responsible* for very little of the decline in crime since the 1990s (Blumstein & Wallman, 2006; Zimring, 2012). Perhaps in response to one or more of these problems, in recent years, there appears to be a shift in attitudes of the public and policymakers regarding the necessity and feasibility of the complete incapacitation for offenders, especially those convicted of minor offenses. For the first time since the "War on Drugs" and the seemingly draconian sentencing policies of the 1980s, optimism that downsizing the prison population is possible is beginning to surface (Drakulich & Kirk, 2016).

Inherent in this shift is the need for suitable alternatives to ensure public safety while building a more just, efficient, and fair response to criminal offending. One approach is sentencing alternatives, which provide judges with an option to require an offender to complete mandatory programs in exchange for a more lenient outcome or a reduced term of incarceration (Engen, Gainey, Crutchfield, & Weis, 2003). For some offenders, these appear to be successful at encouraging desistence from crime because they can better target the needs of offenders, which, in turn, may decrease their proclivity for future offending and increase the chance that they will adopt a prosocial lifestyle (Sevigny, Fuleihan, & Ferdik, 2013).

A promising alternative are initiatives designed specifically to interrupt the cycle of reoffending at reentry. "Reentry," or when an offender returns to his or her home after a period of incarceration, is deemed a critical time in interrupting an offender's lifetime trajectory of offending (Petersilia, 2003). It can be difficult for justice-involved individuals to exit system involvement without support for basic needs such as housing and employment and assistance with gaining further education and basic life skills (Travis & Visher, 2005). Often, substance abuse and other mental health issues make success difficult to achieve (Mallik-Kane & Visher, 2008).

Families of offenders often provide the greatest amount of support and resources for returning offenders during the first year. However, research indicates that the process is extremely stressful for families (Grieb et al., 2014; Naser & Visher, 2006). Further, rearrest and reimprisonment are common scenarios, potentially adding further stress to families (Durose, Cooper, & Snyder, 2014). Children in families with incarcerated parents are at risk for a host of potentially undesirable consequences (Eddy & Poehlmann, 2010), including an increased propensity to commit antisocial behaviors (Murray, Farrington, & Sekol, 2012) and perhaps to become justice-involved themselves (Beaver, 2013; Junger, Schipper, Hesper, Estourgie, & Greene, 2013; van de Weijer, Bijleveld, & Blokland, 2014).

In response to the growing costs of incarceration, fiscal and social, policymakers in Washington State passed the Parenting Sentencing Alternative (aka the "Alternative") in 2010 with the intent of maintaining public safety and reducing the myriad immediate- and long-term costs of incarceration while maintaining and strengthening parent–child bonds. The hope was that these efforts would help interrupt the intergenerational incarceration cycle, not only for parents but also for their children. Here, we describe the creation and implementation of the two prongs of the Parenting Sentencing Alterative (PSA)—the Family Offender Sentencing Alternative (FOSA) and the Community Parenting Alternative (CPA). We then present a preliminary outcome evaluation of the CPA, present a case study to illustrate our findings, and discuss implications for future research.

The Parenting Sentencing Alternative: Development and implementation

In 2010, the Washington State Legislature passed a law titled the PSA, also known as Substitute Senate Bill 6639. The original impetus for the law was fiscal necessity. In 2009, all state agencies were responsible for reducing operating budgets to respond to the diminished economy of the Great Recession. To cut prison costs, Department of Corrections (DOC) staff conceived the idea of creating a sentencing alternative for nonviolent offenders who are parents of minor children.

In collaboration with the Department of Social Health and Services (DSHS), Department of Early Learning (DEL), and judicial court members, the DOC submitted a bill for consideration. The legislation would allow offenders to either avoid prison at the discretion of a judge or transfer from prison up to 12 months early on electronic home monitoring (EHM) and serve the remainder of their prison sentence at home with their children. The goal was for parents to learn active parenting skills as well as the ability to balance the responsibilities of parenthood and community living rather than remaining in total confinement. The bill became law on June 10, 2010, and approximately 6 weeks later, the review committed selected the first offender for participation in the program.

Program development

The law created eight new positions: one program administrator, one program manager, and six community corrections officers (CCOs; often referred to elsewhere as probation or parole officers). The six CCOs were necessary to allow a specialized caseload and permit participation across Washington State. Over time, the program has grown, and eight CCOs are required. The program administrator has a social work background and more than 20 years of experience in corrections. Other staff hired for the program seemed eager to embrace a less traditional, or strict, form of community corrections, and turn to one with a greater emphasis on strength-building and positive approaches to problem solving.

Together, the new program staff team developed the program goals, mission, and values during the 3-day training session. Program development goals included placing children of offenders at the apex of every decision and making family reunification decisions that would allow participation in the Alternative. To achieve this goal, the DOC built partnerships with other state agencies specializing in family and child safety to ensure all decisions are in the "best interests" of the offenders' children. In Washington State, this is defined as follows: "The best interests of the child are served by a parenting arrangement that best maintains a child's emotional growth, health and stability, and physical care" (Dissolution Proceedings-Legal Separation Policy, 2007).

Staff members also recognized the need for assistance and partnerships to better understand family dynamics. The state Children's Administration (i.e., the state child welfare system) provided training to staff in social work principles for case management and created regional contacts as needed for individual cases. A partnership with the state DEL influenced the team and resulted in a focus on a "strengthening families" model. The model uses five protective factors to strengthen and sustain families: social and emotional competence of children, knowledge of child development and parenting, concrete support in times of need, social connections, and parental resilience. Over the years, the DEL has provided ongoing training to staff on topics such as family dynamics, adverse childhood experiences, and ages and stages of development.

Last, it was critical to create a highly structured alternative because some offenders would be transferring from institutionalized confinement to their homes on electronic monitoring. Staff designed a program that used skills training paired with progressive discipline to help offenders learn to organize their time and prioritize needs; build "soft skills" such as communication, budgeting, relationships, and emotional management; and receive immediate consequences when they did not meet expectations.

In sum, the structure of the Alternative is a combination of core correctional and social work practices within an interagency-supported framework designed to meet the challenges faced by offenders and their families during reentry. DOC uses a structured strengths-based approach with offenders and families to determine what works best for a given individual in the program and to help him or her succeed, in the short run and over the long run.

Program eligibility and implementation

By law, team staff members are responsible for the implementation of both options of the PSA: the FOSA and the CPA. While the premises behind the two options are the same, there are some substantial differences in eligibility and rigor, especially regarding level of contact with CCOs. Before participation in FOSA, offenders are not incarcerated for their current conviction. Participation in one option of the PSA does not preclude an offender from participating in the other.

The Family Offender Sentencing Alternative

The FOSA is a court-based alternative. It provides judges with the option to waive a prison sentence if they deem it appropriate and to impose 12 months of community custody in lieu of prison. FOSA offenders must meet specific eligibility criteria defined by the law (see Table 1).

To ensure offender eligibility when considering this option at the time of sentencing, the court may order the DOC to conduct a chemical dependency screening and/or a Risk Assessment Report (RAR) (Washington State Department of Corrections, 2014). The CCO interviews the defendant, conducts a home investigation and checks references to gain an understanding of the defendant's current circumstances. Simultaneously, DOC sends release of

Table 1. Parenting Sentencing Alternative Eligibility Criteria.

Criterion	CPA	FOSA
Sentence range	Longer than 1 year	Longer than 1 year
Offense level	No current conviction for a felony sex or violent crime	No prior or current conviction for a felony sex or violent crime
Citizenship	Not subject to deportation order during period of sentence	Not currently subject to deportation and does not become subject to deportation during period of sentence
Children's welfare	Parent agrees to sign release of information regarding prior or current child welfare cases DOC determines placement with parent is in the best interest of the child	Parent agrees to sign release of information regarding prior or current child welfare cases
Custody	Has proven, established, ongoing, and substantial relationship with his or her minor child that existed prior to the commission of the current offense *or* is a legal guardian of a child who was under the age of 18 at the time of the current offense	Has physical custody of his or her minor child or is a legal guardian or custodian with physical custody of a child under the age of 18 at the time of current offense

information forms signed by the offender to Children's Administration and the DSHS to obtain child welfare history as well as parental substance abuse or mental health treatment histories to validate information reported by offenders during the RAR assessment.

In the end, the court makes a discretionary decision based on all of the factors of the case, including offense severity, suitability of the alternative for the offender, and victim, child, public, and offender safety. If the court determines FOSA is an appropriate alternative, the judge waives the prison sentence and imposes 12 months of community custody supervision. In doing so, the law permits the court to impose conditions including (but not limited to) parenting classes, chemical dependency treatment, mental health treatment, vocational training, offender change programs, and life skills classes. Stipulations for participation vary by offender. The DOC can also impose additional conditions, as long as those conditions have a nexus to the criminal behavior and community risk.

Once the program is active, the law requires that CCOs provide quarterly progress reports for each offender to the court. The court may also require an offender to appear at any time for a progress report or if a violation has occurred. If the offender fails to make reasonable progress while on the alternative or violates the conditions of supervision, the court schedules a hearing at their discretion to address the issue. Sanctions vary at the discretion of the court as the law does not define guidelines for standards of progressive discipline. If an offender consistently fails to meet the conditions required to retain community supervision status, the court will "revoke" the alternative sentence order and impose the original prison sentence. The offender will receive credit for any time served in confinement but not for any participation in the alternative sentencing program.

The Community Parenting Alternative

In contrast, the CPA is a prison-based alternative. It allows an offender who is currently incarcerated to be transferred to his or her home on EHM for up to the last year of their sentence if the offender has a minor child. It must be in the best interests of the child to be reunited with the parent. CPA participants must meet much of the same criteria for FOSA, with a few modifications and extensions (see Table 1). Program conditions differ from FOSA in that they are more rigorous. The offenders are more intensely supervised and must be on EHM because they are inmates in the community.

To ensure offender eligibility when considering this option to release an offender from prison, the DOC completes a "transfer plan" containing information about the offender's convictions, work programs, treatment, drug history, visitation history, infraction history, and family history and an assessment interview. The program manager then develops a plan for the offender and ensures it is compatible with all legal criteria and policy requirements.

Transfer plans are referred to the CCOs who conduct a home investigation. This investigation is intended to get the "sponsor" (i.e., the offender's family) engaged. They must be dedicated to supporting the interests of the children and demonstrate willingness to collaborate with the DOC to provide resources and opportunities for returning offenders to be "present parents." Parents must be clean, sober, and able to prioritize their children in daily decisions.

The CCO explains to the sponsor the requirements of participation. These include no weapons, alcohol, or drugs in the home and participation in family dinners at a table without the distraction of television or other electronic devices. Further, the offender must read to their children or assist them with homework for at least 20 minutes per day, depending on the child's age. The family must have a dedicated landline telephone to enable EHM. However, there is no cost for this line to the sponsor. This was intentionally included as part of the bill by the legislature to prevent an economic disparity from determining who could participate.

With the sponsor ready to engage, the transfer plan is then used by the multidisciplinary screening committee to determine whether the offender should be selected for participation in the alternative. The committee is composed of professionals who are child welfare experts and other stakeholders who have an interest in children, families, and offenders reentering communities. If the committee recommends the offender be selected for participation, the law requires approval of the plan by the assistant secretary of community corrections; the secretary of DOC then gives final approval of the plan.

While participating in CPA, offenders must account for every hour of their day. All activities at home and in the community must be verified, including attendance at school, work, or other appointments. Every daily activity must be preapproved by the CCO. Offenders are not allowed to obtain employment during their initial participation in the program. This requirement is to ensure they are spending as much time as possible with their children, reestablishing bonds, building positive relationships, and fulfilling the conditions of their release. Offenders speak with their CCOs on a daily basis, and CCOs conduct frequent home inspections to ensure compliance.

Sanctions are more likely for CPA participants compared with FOSA participants. CPA has higher levels of accountability because participants are DOC inmates completing their prison sentence in the community on EHM rather than in prison. While on this alternative, DOC addresses any violations of rules; violation of rules will result in the offender's return to prison, with a loss of good time, to serve the remainder of the current sentence.

Method

Research question

Because the PSA was created and funded by the Washington State Legislature, administrators at the DOC were required to assess preliminary outcomes and report back to the lawmakers who wrote the bill. To achieve this goal, researchers at the Washington State Institute for Criminal Justice agreed to undertake a phased evaluation. In 2012, the first analysis was completed, namely an impact evaluation to measure outcomes of the CPA option during the first 2 years of implementation. The results of that evaluation are presented here. The primary research question to examine the impact of the CPA was as follows: Will offenders who participated in the CPA have significantly reduced felony recidivism in the first 2 years after release compared with a similar control group of offenders who did not participate?

Data collection

Data were gathered from routinely collected DOC administrative records and offender responses to a risk-needs-responsivity tool. The tool included the Adult Static Risk Assessment (ASRA) (Drake, 2014) and the Offender Needs Assessment (ONA); they are collectively called the STRONG risk assessment (Desmarais & Singh, 2013). The ASRA has a moderate predictive accuracy with AUCs for all risk levels and offense types at greater than 0.7 (Barnoski & Drake, 2007). The first author received deidentified data for analysis after obtaining institutional review board approval at Washington State University and the Washington State DOC.

Sample

The evaluation sample frame consisted of all offenders in Washington State who were statutorily eligible for selection as a CPA participant between 2008 and 2012 ($N = 393$). A historic comparison group was created of offenders who were released between 2008 and 2010 who would have been eligible for the alternative had it been available ($n = 334$). The experimental group consisted of all offenders who were accepted for participation in the CPA and were released between 2010 and 2012 ($n = 59$). Of the 107 accepted for CPA on the date of analysis, 46 had successfully completed the program, 13 were terminated before completion, 44 were still participating, and 4 were participants in both alternatives. These dual participants were removed from the analyses because the focus of the analyses was outcomes due to CPA alone. Demographic information about participants is provided in Table 2.

Variables

The *dependent variable*, recidivism, was defined as any felony offense committed by an offender within 24 months of being at risk in the community that resulted in a Washington State conviction ("0" = no, "1" = yes). The *independent variable*, participation status, was operationalized as any participation in the CPA ("0" = no, "1" = yes), using the intent to treat standard of inclusion (Guo & Fraser, 2010). All offenders who were admitted to CPA were included in the analysis, not just those who successfully completed the program.

Suitability for predictor variables to include in the match was determined first by selecting theoretically relevant predictors from the more than 180 items included in the ASRA and ONA. Second, predictors that could be a significant source of bias between the participant and comparison groups, and therefore should be controlled for in the impact evaluation, were identified by using a backward stepwise regression with significance set at $p = 0.1$ (Guo & Fraser, 2010). In the end, the following *control variables* were included in the propensity score match: age at current offense ("0" = 18–29, "1" = 30–39, "2" = 40–60 or older), gender ("0" = male, "1" = female), race ("0" = not White, "1" = White), risk level ("0" = low, "1" = moderate, "2" = high), education level ("0" = 11th grade or less, "1" = high school diploma or GED, "2" = more than GED or high school), longest legal employment ("0" = longer than 1 year, "1" = less than 1 year), current incarceration length ("0" = longer than 1 year, "1" = less than 1 year), number of programs completed while incarcerated ("0" = none, "1" = 1 or 2, "2" = 3 or more), juvenile felony conviction ("0" = no, "1" = yes), mental health problem ever ("0" = no, "1" = yes), and substance abuse problem ever ("0" = no, "1" = yes).

Table 2. Propensity Score Matching Descriptives.

	Prematching (n = 393)			Postmatching (n = 116)		
Measure	Comparison, % (n = 334)	Participants, % (n = 59)	STD Difference	Comparison, % (n = 58)	Participants, % (n = 58)	STD Difference
Female	39.2	88.1***	0.72	74.1	87.9 †	0.17
Age at current offense (yr)						
18–29	36.2	50.8 †	0.33	46.6	50.0	0.07
30–39	41.6	37.3	0.11	41.4	37.9	0.08
40–60 or older	22.2	11.9	0.59	12.1	12.1	0.00
White	74.6	78.0	0.04	79.3	77.6	0.02
Risk level						
Low	11.1	25.4**	0.74	19.0	24.1	0.24
Moderate	25.7	27.1	0.05	27.6	27.6	0.00
High	63.2	47.5	0.28	53.4	48.3	0.10
Highest grade completed						
11th grade or less	37.4	25.4**	0.38	29.3	25.9	0.12
GED or high school (HS)	40.4	32.2	0.22	34.5	32.8	0.17
Higher than GED or HS	22.2	42.4**	0.60	36.2	41.4	0.13
Incarcerated less than 1 year	77.2	50.8***	0.40	69.0	51.7†	0.28
Juvenile felony conviction	8.4	16.9*	0.66	10.3	17.2	0.50
Number of minor children						
1	44.0	35.6	0.22	37.9	36.2	0.04
≥2	56.0	64.4	0.14	62.1	63.8	0.02
Mental health problem	59.9	47.5 †	0.23	46.6	46.6	0.00
Substance abuse problem	61.4	33.9***	0.56	46.6	34.5	0.29
Employed less than 1 year	46.4	47.5	0.02	41.4	48.3	0.15
Programs completed						
None	31.7	37.3	0.16	27.6	37.9	0.31
1–2	37.4	30.5	0.20	39.7	31.0	0.24
≥3	30.8	32.2	0.04	32.8	31.0	0.05

Note. †$p < .1$, *$p < .05$, **$p < .01$, ***$p < .001$.

Comparison group development

A propensity score match was created to reduce observable bias between the participant and comparison groups before comparing recidivistic outcomes. Participants can be matched on a propensity score to create a comparison group when randomized trials are not possible, unethical, or illegal (Guo & Fraser, 2010; Rosenbaum & Rubin, 1983). This decreases the likelihood that results of the analysis are due to chance, rather than to the effects of the intervention of interest. For this analysis, the propensity score was calculated without replacement using a 1:1 nearest-neighbor greedy match with a caliper of 0.25 (Guo & Fraser, 2010). That is, each participant was matched statistically to one offender in the comparison group by using the composite score of their location in the propensity score within an acceptable range based on the control variables predicting participation in the CPA.

The two groups were compared on each predictor before and after the propensity score match to determine whether observable bias still existed between the two groups after the match. Significant bivariate differences were calculated using crosstabs with Pearson's χ^2 (see Table 2 for prematch and postmatch bivariate comparisons). A measure of sensitivity, the area under the curve (AUC) statistic, revealed that the match decreased the differences between the two groups (before AUC = 0.890, 95% confidence interval [CI] 0.846–0.933, $p < .001$; after AUC = 0.685, 95% CI 0.589–0.781, $p < .001$). However, the AUC postmatch would ideally be 0.50, suggesting each offender had an equal chance of being in the participant or control group; no observable bias unduly influenced the results (Rice & Harris, 2005). Additionally, there were six standardized differences; this is a measure of effect size and exceeded 0.20. This indicates the match did not achieve ideal balance between the two groups.

Before the propensity score match, there were seven significant bivariate differences between the participant and comparison groups. The groups differed on gender, education level, length of incarceration, presence of a juvenile felony conviction, and presence of a problem with substance abuse. There were also two comparisons that neared but did not achieve statistical significance: mental health problem and age at release from prison. In brief, compared with the control group, participants were significantly more likely to be female, younger, lower risk, and better educated and to have been incarcerated longer and have a juvenile felony conviction they were less likely to have a mental health or substance abuse problem. After the match, only two bivariate comparisons neared significance: gender [$\chi^2 = 3.59(1)$, $p = .058$] and incarceration length [$\chi^2 = 3.60(1)$, $p = .058$]. None were significant at $p < .05$.

Analyses

Outcomes were compared using crosstabs with the χ^2 statistic (see Table 3) to determine whether the CPA reduced the likelihood that an offender who participated would be convicted of a new felony within 2 years compared with offenders who were similarly situated and did not participate.

Table 3. Felony Recidivism by Study Group.

	Year 1			Year 2		
Outcome	Comparison, %	Participant, %	OR	Comparison, %	Participant, %	OR
Any felony	8.6	0.0†	0.00	17.2	5.2*	0.26

Note. †$p < .1$, *$p < .05$. OR, odds ratio.

Results

Two years after release, offenders who participated in the CPA were significantly less likely to be convicted of a new felony [$\chi^2 = 4.24(1)$, $p < .05$]. Moreover, being a CPA participant reduced the odds of being convicted of a new felony 2 years after release by 71%. As a point of further comparison, the average rate of recidivism after 2 years among offenders released in Washington State between 1991 and 2006 was between 8.8% and 13.3% (Evans, 2010).

Discussion

CPA participants were significantly less likely to recidivate after 2 years of release than were a matched group of offenders who did not participate. Conceptually, this finding is unsurprising. Reentry is challenging for offenders (Durose et al., 2014; Petersilia, 2003) and their families (Grieb et al., 2014). Support is essential for returning offenders, and the holistic services provided by this program are quite encompassing and include a network of partnerships (including community service providers and child welfare) designed to help ensure success. Such partnerships have been recommended by criminologists to ensure that scarce resources are directed to the communities and people most in need (Lutze, Johnson, Clear, Latessa, & Slate, 2012). Additionally, the use of graduated sanctions and a focus on a strength-building approach to community corrections may be protective for offenders and CCOs (Drapela & Lutze, 2009; Lutze et al., 2012).

This study provides an important contribution, albeit a preliminary one, to the literature. While there are a number of parenting programs for prisoners designed to mitigate the potential risks of parental incarceration (Eddy & Poehlmann, 2010), this is the first to the researchers' knowledge to combine these programs with services and resources during reentry through community supervision while involving the child heavily in the offender's daily life. The lessons learned from this pioneering sentencing alternative ultimately will assist policymakers and administrators who desire to replicate this program in other states.

The results should be interpreted with caution due to the limitations of the research design and analyses. An important item missing from this analysis is an assessment of program fidelity and a consideration of fidelity in the outcome evaluation. The rigorous documentation of program elements in each case would be beneficial. This would enable an examination of key issues such as how differing amounts of program resources and supervision relates to outcomes, how consistently the program's resources and time are devoted to each offender, and what impact levels of participation had on the outcomes of the offenders who were terminated and did not successfully complete the program.

Further, the analyses consider only one outcome of participation in the CPA—recidivism. There are several other desired outcomes of the program stated in the program goals and objectives, including building sustainable families, reducing intergenerational incarceration, reducing duplicative services, and maintaining family and community safety. Reducing offending after release is only one small component of the program. Future research is planned that will examine changes needed over time after participation, the impact of the program on the offender's family members, and the effect of the program on reducing intergenerational incarceration.

Finally, the propensity score match was not as strong as desired to be considered reliable. Postmatch, the standardized differences should be no greater than 0.2 (Rice & Harris, 2005), yet six of the predictor variables exceeded this standard. For these results to be reliable, a greater common support region between the two groups is needed (Guo & Fraser, 2010). Further, although 3 years of outcomes are considered standard to determine whether a program is reducing recidivism (Durose et al., 2014; Petersilia, 2003), this analysis, completed with available data in 2013, included only 2 years of outcomes. In short, multiple replications of these findings, using more rigorous research designs, are needed to overcome these limitations.

Nonetheless, these initial results show promise and are worthy of consideration as the CPA is, to the researchers' knowledge, the first of its kind in the nation. The limitations inherent in this analysis provide lessons for replication in other states, and forthcoming analyses will determine the reliability of these results. Fortunately, replication, and the opportunity for further outcome studies, is already in action. In Washington State, analyses of the FOSA program are under way, as are additional analyses of new CPA participants. Further, the state of Oregon recently passed legislation establishing a PSA on a pilot basis in selected counties. Collaborative plans are being made to jointly evaluate efforts across the two states.

While necessary, program descriptions and numerical research findings are not sufficient to capture what happens when an alternative sentence is applied. Thus, in conclusion, we present a brief case study to illustrate the experience from the perspective of one participant who was involved in the CPA. We will refer to the participant as Gina.

Case study

Gina was 39 years of age when selected to participate in the CPA. She had previously been incarcerated four times. Her most recent conviction resulted in a sentence of 8 years for several crimes including burglary, identify theft, drug possession, and possession of stolen property. As an unemployed methamphetamine addict, she was motivated to commit crimes to survive. Gina had five children when she was sentenced to prison, three boys and two girls, who were between the ages of 5 and 15. Only two were still minors during the last 12 months of her sentence when she became eligible to participate in the CPA. While incarcerated, Gina was saddened by the strained relationships between herself and her children. Although most of them visited her in prison, the visits were hardly conducive to heartfelt discussion or shared private moments. Outside of the institutional visits, Gina had phone contact with her children but experienced difficulties addressing issues due to the time limits for conversations. During her incarceration, Gina had avoided dealing with the challenges in her relationships. This regret and sadness were strong motivations for Gina to apply for the CPA and to succeed during her supervision.

Gina felt fragmented during the first 3 months in the CPA. She commented on how difficult it was to meet competing commitments, such as treatment, sober support meetings, cognitive behavioral classes, keeping up with her children's school schedule, preparing meals, daily hygiene, household chores, and assisting her children with their homework. She found herself grateful for the structure of the CPA, which required that she establish a schedule to meet the needs of her family.

Gina had burned bridges with most of her family due to her behavior before incarceration, so she had nowhere to live when released. She was able to secure housing at a clean and sober complex that allowed children as part of the program. Housing was one of the needed supports recognized by the screening committee when Gina was approved to participate, so she received housing assistance from the CPA to improve her chances of being successful.

Gina reported that the support of her CCO was essential. Her CCO attempted to warn Gina about some of the challenges she would encounter once released, including the difficulties adjusting to a greater level of contact with her children. Once the realities of the program set in, Gina was glad for the required daily phone calls and frequent in-person contact with her CCO. During these calls, the CCO spent a lot of time providing counsel regarding how Gina could best meet her children's needs. As Gina progressed through the program, she continued to contact her CCO frequently, even when not required. Additionally, as part of the CPA, the CCO worked with community service providers to ensure Gina became familiar with the resources available to her. While providing this positive support, the CCO also ensured accountability by using progressive levels of discipline. Examples of this included restricting Gina to her home if she was late and written reports explaining the consequences if Gina did not follow her plan.

It has been 3 years since Gina graduated from the CPA. She made remarkable changes in her life during and after the program. Gina is currently employed as a caregiver in the healthcare field. She has health benefits and earns a wage that provides a nice standard of living for herself and her children. She resolved her legal financial obligations and was able to get a driver's license and purchase a reliable car.

Gina was able to build a solid relationship with her children; these relationships were most important to her. She built trust by being available to them when they needed her. The healthy habits she built during the CPA related to organization and consistency; this translated into more time with her children. Every day Gina is thankful that she was able to spend the last few years of her youngest children's childhoods with them. She also reports that her older children have become more interested in building a relationship with her now that they see the progress she has made. They no longer fear they will be a second priority to addiction.

In conclusion, although Gina often felt like giving up and going back to prison, she began to understand that the CPA was difficult but worth it. Rather than experience reentry alone or return to the same environment she had left when incarcerated (which she may have done if she had been released directly from prison), Gina leaned up the support of her CCO, embraced the structure of the alternative, and accepted the resources offered to her. This changed not only her ability to sustain herself and improve her relationships with her family but also how she viewed herself and her role as a mother. It would have been impossible for Gina to reach these milestones if she had not also mastered the skills of consistency, resilience, and reliability during her participation in the CPA. With these, she was able to succeed during reentry and beyond.

References

Barnoski, R., & Drake, E. K. (2007). *Washington's Offender Accountability Act*. Olympia, WA: Washington State Department of Corrections.

Beaver, K. M. (2013). The familial concentration and transmission of crime. *Criminal Justice & Behavior, 40*(2), 139–155. doi:10.1177/0093854812449405

Blumstein, A., & Wallman, J. (2006). The recent rise and fall of American violence. In *In The crime drop in America* (2nd ed., pp. 1–12). New York, NY: Cambridge University Press.

Clear, T. R. (2007). *Imprisoning communities: How mass incarceration makes disadvantaged neighborhoods worse*. New York, NY: Oxford University Press.

Clear, T. R., & Frost, N. A. (2014). *The punishment imperative: The rise and failure of mass incarceration in America*. New York, NY: New York University Press.

Currie, E. (2013). *Crime and punishment in America*. New York, NY: Picador.

Desmarais, S., & Singh, J. P. (2013). *Assessment instruments validation and implemented in correctional settings in the United States: An empirical guide*. New York, NY: Council of State Government Justice Center.

Dissolution Proceedings-Legal Separation Policy. (2007). Pub. L. No. RCW 26.09.002. Revised Code of Washington. Retrieved from http://apps.leg.wa.gov/rcw/default.aspx?cite=26.09.002

Drake, E. (2014). *Predicting criminal recidivism: A systematic review of offender risk assessments in Washington State*. Olympia, WA: Washington State Institute for Public Policy. Retrieved from http://www.wsipp.wa.gov

Drakulich, K. M., & Kirk, E. M. (2016). Public opinion and criminal justice reform. *Criminology & Public Policy, 15*(1), 171–177. doi:10.1111/1745-9133.12186

Drapela, L. A., & Lutze, F. E. (2009). Innovation in community corrections and probation officers' fears of being sued: Implementing neighborhood-based supervision in Spokane, Washington. *Journal of Contemporary Criminal Justice, 25*(4), 364–383. doi:10.1177/1043986209344549

Durose, M. R., Cooper, A. D., & Snyder, H. N. (2014). *Recidivism of prisoners released in 30 states in 2005: Patterns from 2005 to 2010*. Washington, DC: Bureau of Justice Statistics. Retrieved from http://www.bjs.gov/content/pub/pdf/rprts05p0510.pdf

Eddy, J. M., & Poehlmann, J. (2010). *Children of incarcerated parents: A handbook for researchers and practitioners*. Washington, D.C: Urban Institute Press.

Engen, R. L., Gainey, R. R., Crutchfield, R. D., & Weis, J. G. (2003). Discretion and disparity under sentencing guidelines: The role of departures and structured sentencing alternatives. *Criminology, 41*(1), 99–130. doi:10.1111/j.1745-9125.2003.tb00983.x

Evans, M. (2010). *Recidivism revisited*. Olympia, WA: Washington State Department Corrections. Retrieved from http://www.doc.wa.bov/aboutdc/measurestatistics/doc/RecidivismRevisited.pdf

Grieb, S. M. D., Crawford, A., Fields, J., Smith, H., Harris, R., & Matson, P. (2014). "The stress will kill you": Prisoner reentry as experienced by family members and the urgent need for support services. *Journal of Health Care for the Poor and Underserved, 25*(3), 1183–1200. doi:10.1353/hpu.2014.0118

Guo, S., & Fraser, M. W. (2010). *Propensity score analysis: Statistical methods and applications*. Los Angeles, CA: Sage Publications, Inc.

Junger, J., Schipper, R., Hesper, F., Estourgie, V., & Greene, M. (2013). Parental criminality, family violence and intergenerational transmission of crime within a birth cohort. *European Journal on Criminal Policy and Research, 19*(2), 117–133. doi:10.1007/s10610-012-9193-z

Lutze, F. E., Johnson, W. W., Clear, T. R., Latessa, E. J., & Slate, R. N. (2012). The future of community corrections is now: Stop dreaming and take action. *Journal of Contemporary Criminal Justice, 28*(1), 42–59. doi:10.1177/1043986211432193

Mallik-Kane, K., & Visher, C. A. (2008). *Health and prisoner reentry: How physical, mental, and substance abuse conditions shape the process of reintegration.* Washington, DC: Urban Institute Justice Policy Center.

Murray, J., Farrington, D. P., & Sekol, I. (2012). Children's antisocial behavior, mental health, drug use, and educational performance after parental incarceration: A systematic review and meta-analysis. *Psychological Bulletin, 138*(2), 175–210. doi:10.1037/a0026407

Naser, R. L., & Visher, C. A. (2006). Family members' experiences with incarceration and reentry. *Western Criminology Review, 7*(2), 20–31.

Petersilia, J. (2003). *When prisoners come home: Parole and prisoner reentry.* New York, NY: Oxford University Press.

Reiman, J. H., & Leighton, P. (2010). *The rich get richer and the poor get prison: Ideology, class, and criminal justice* (9th ed.). Boston, MA: Allyn & Bacon.

Rice, M. E., & Harris, G. T. (2005). Comparing effect sizes in follow-up studies: ROC area, Cohen's d, and r. *Law and Human Behavior, 29*(5), 615–620. doi:10.1007/s10979-005-6832-7

Rosenbaum, P. R., & Rubin, D. B. (1983). The central role of the propensity score in observational studies for causal effects. *Biometrika, 70*, 41–55.

Sevigny, E. L., Fuleihan, B. K., & Ferdik, F. V. (2013). Do drug courts reduce the use of incarceration?: A meta-analysis. *Journal of Criminal Justice, 41*(6), 416–425. doi:10.1016/j.jcrimjus.2013.06.005

Travis, J., & Visher, C. (2005). *Prisoner reentry and crime in America.* New York, NY: Cambridge University Press.

van de Weijer, S. G. A., Bijleveld, C. C. J. H., & Blokland, A. A. J. (2014). The intergenerational transmission of violent offending. *Journal of Family Violence, 29*, 109–118. doi:10.1007/s10896-013-9565-2

Walker, S., Spohn, C., & DeLone, M. (2012). *The color of justice: Race, ethnicity, and crime in America.* Belmont, CA: Wadsworth.

Washington State Department of Corrections. (2014). *DOC policy 320.010.* Retrieved from http://www.doc.wa.gov/information/policies/files/320010.pdf

Zimring, F. E. (2012). *The great American crime decline.* New York, NY: Oxford University Press.

The Moderating Effect of Living with a Child Before Incarceration on Postrelease Outcomes Related to a Prison-Based Parent Management Training Program

Bert O. Burraston, PhD, and J. Mark Eddy, PhD

ABSTRACT
With the rapid growth in incarceration in the United States over the past few decades came dramatic growth in the number of the incarcerated parents with at least one minor child. Parental incarceration places extra stresses and strains on families and children. Almost all of those incarcerated will eventually be released. However, the majority of those released from prison will be rearrested within a year. Finding interventions that can decrease the likelihood of returning to crime and to incarceration are of utmost importance. Using a social bond theory framework, the authors examine the moderating effect of living with a child before incarceration on program outcomes related to a prison-based parent management training program. A significant effect was found. Implications for these findings are discussed for future research and practice.

The dramatic and well-documented growth in incarceration in the United States during the past several decades has also resulted in a dramatic growth in the number of incarcerated parents (Travis, Western, & Redburn, 2014). The majority of those who are incarcerated today are a parent of at least one minor child, estimated at 53% of men and 61% of women (Maruschak, Glaze, & Mumola, 2010; Glaze & Maruschak, 2010; Mumola, 2000). Over time, this means that a large number of children are affected by parental incarceration. For example, Western and Wildeman (2009) estimated that between 1980 and 2000, the number of children whose fathers were incarcerated grew from 350,000 to 1.2 million. Further, Murphey and Cooper (2015) estimated that 5 million children have had at least one custodial parent incarcerated in jail or prison at some point in their childhood. They point out, however, that this estimate does not include nonresidential parents and therefore is a substantial underestimation of the total number of children who have had at least one parent incarcerated at some point during their childhood.

The majority of those who are incarcerated will be released from prison (Mumola, 2000; Travis, 2000). Thus, the massive growth in incarceration has also led to a massive growth in offenders being released from prison and reentering society. For example, in 2014 in the United States, federal and state prisons combined released 636,300 inmates back to their communities (Carson, 2015). Such a number, again, substantially underestimates the number of children affected by incarceration that year as it does not include the number of men and women released from their local jails.

Reentering society and successfully engaging in life on the outside are not easy. One illustration of this is the significant number of people who return to lock-up after release. In this regard, most individuals who return home will be rearrested within 5 years (Durose, Cooper, & Snyder, 2014; Langan & Levin, 2002). In a recent U.S. Department of Justice report on recidivism, 28% were rearrested within the first 6 months, 58% were rearrested within the first year, and 77% were rearrested within 5 years of release (Durose et al., 2014). To interrupt this cycle of incarceration, there is a dire need for the field to develop effective ways to prepare, support and assist offenders in the adoption and practice of prosocial lifestyles as they leave prison and reenter their communities.

Issues regarding reentry

There are many issues that those reentering society face including, but not limited to, finding housing, finding a job, reconnecting with family and friends, avoiding substance abuse, paying off fines and fees associated with the criminal justice system, and complying with the terms of community supervision (e.g., Braman, 2004; Geller, Garfinkel, & Western, 2011; Grinstead, Faigeles, Bancroft, & Zack, 2001; Nelson, Deess, & Allen, 1999). Most people who are released initially end up living with family or friends, but this is not always possible because of relationship strains related to factors such as their criminal and substance abuse histories, and the consequences of such, as well as new issues such as restrictions on where they can reside. For example, the partner and children of an incarcerated father are at an increased risk for homelessness during his stay in prison, so there might not even be a home to which to return (Foster & Hagan, 2007; Geller & Walker Franklin, 2014; Wildeman, 2014). Even if their family still resides in their original home, for those fathers who were married, incarceration increases the likelihood of separation and divorce (Lopoo & Western, 2005). Along these lines, Turney and Wildeman (2013) found an increased likelihood that a mother, whether or not married, will end her relationship with the incarcerated father and form a new relationship with a nonincarcerated man.

Across a variety of studies, there are a number of factors that have been found to be associated with recidivism. In particular, number of prior arrests, total years spent in prison, gender (men), age (younger), and mental health problems are associated with higher risk of rearrests (e.g., Gendreau, Little, & Goggin, 1996; Ndrecka, 2014; Schmidt & White, 1989). Beyond these individual risk factors, and of much interest to the criminal justice system across the decades, connection to family is a protective factor that appears to reduce the risk of recidivism (e.g., Bales & Mears, 2008). The relation between connection to family and outcomes related to a prison-based parent management training program is the focus of this article.

Theoretical foundations

For some parents, incarceration can serve as a positive turning point in their life, a time of rehabilitation, and a time when needed treatment for substance abuse, anger management, and other problems is provided (Edin, Nelson, & Paranal, 2004). Further, prison can be a time a parent earns a GED and/or improves his or her jobs skills through employment programs. Less common is having prison serve as a time to address issues related to the family life of a parent. There are theoretical reasons to consider this, too, as an important activity during a prison sentence.

Hirschi's (2002) social bond theory, also known as social control theory, is one of the most prominent criminological theories to link families with the development and maintenance of criminal behaviors. According to Hirschi, it is social bonds that play a key role in preventing people from engaging in illegal behavior, primarily due to fear that such behavior will damage their relationship with friends, parents/family members, neighbors, teachers, employers, and others. Social bonds contain four major elements: social attachments, commitment, involvement, and belief. Of social attachments, the attachments of parent to child and child to parent are thought to be the most important. These attachments are hypothesized to prevent many adolescents from engaging in criminal behavior and to have long-term effects on desistance from crime during adulthood. Further, using a life-course paradigm, Laub and Sampson (2001) found that family-related events, such as marriage, are key turning points in terms of desisting from crime (Sampson & Laub, 1993; Laub & Sampson, 2001). For women, they found that having a child is the number one turning point related to desistance.

From this theoretical viewpoint, one of the key dangers of incarceration in terms of long-term outcomes for a parent and his or her child is that it weakens parent–child attachments and husband–wife (or committed couple) attachments, leaving the parent and the child with weaker societal bonds and thus putting both in positions where they are likely to engage in future criminal behavior. For example, Turney and Wildeman (2013) found strong negative relations between parental incarceration and parent–child engagement, shared responsibility in parenting, and cooperation in parenting.

The majority of incarcerated parents have a minor child (Maruschak, Glaze, & Mumola, 2010), and thus simply having a child is not sufficient to deter an individual from further criminal behavior. Beyond family events alone, Hughes (1998) identified six turning points that contributed to desistance from criminal behavior: respect and concern for children, incarceration, fear of physical harm, time to contemplate, support, and modeling. It would be very difficult for a parent and child to bond properly if the parent has not learned respect and concern for children, so a prison-based parenting intervention program that teaches about children's needs as well as respect and concern for children, either in tandem or followed by the opportunity to connect with a child, could lead to reductions in recidivism.

Parent management training (PMT; Forgatch & Martinez, 1999) is a cognitive-behavioral intervention that was originally designed to reduce child and adolescent antisocial behavior in outpatient clinical populations. In terms of efficacy, PMT has met the stringent criterion of being "well established" (e.g., Brestan & Eyberg, 1998). During the past few decades, a variety of evidence-based PMT programs have been adapted for nonclinical settings (Reid, Patterson, & Snyder, 2002; Webster-Stratton & Taylor, 2001). The five primary skill sets taught in most PMT programs are parental positive involvement, parental encouragement, noncoercive and nonaversive discipline (prosocial discipline), child monitoring and supervision, and family problem-solving skills (Eddy et al., 2008). PMT is intended to provide parents with the background information and practice needed to know which parenting skill to use and when, based on factors such as the child's age, development, temperament, and the situation.

PMT is grounded in social interaction learning theory (SLT; Patterson, Reid, & Dishion, 1992). Within SLT, coercive family processes and inept discipline practices play key roles in the development of antisocial and criminal behavior across the lifespan (Patterson, Capaldi, & Bank, 1991). One of the major findings that led to positing SLT is that early failures in discipline, consistent child noncompliance, problematic social attachments (including between parent and child), and low levels of social skills appear to set in motion and continue the development of antisocial and criminal behaviors (Patterson, 1982; Patterson et al., 1991; Reid & Eddy, 1997). SLT emphasizes that development throughout the life course happens through interactions between prior dispositions, the learning history of an individual, and the current environments (and individuals within those environments) to which he/she is exposed (Cairns & Cairns, 1994; Caspi & Elder, 1988; Hetherington & Baltes, 1988; Magnusson & Torestad, 1993; Rutter, 1989). There is a significant body of research that shows PMT can prevent or interrupt negative parent–child interactions related to child antisocial behavior (Brestan & Eyberg, 1998; Reid et al., 2002; Webster-Stratton & Taylor, 2001). What has not been tested sufficiently is whether PMT can act as a turning point for incarcerated parents.

The purpose of this article is to conduct a preliminary test of PMT as a turning point through a test of moderation of the effect of a prison-based PMT program, *Parenting Inside Out* (PIO), on 1-year postrelease arrests using data from a randomized controlled trial. Five of the six turning points of desisting from criminal behavior identified by Hughes (1998) are associated with PIO, namely respect and concern for children, incarceration, time to contemplate, support, and modeling. PIO (Eddy, Kjellstrand, Martinez, & Newton, 2010; Eddy et al., 2008; Schiffman, Eddy, Martinez, Leve, & Newton, 2008) was designed for delivery to groups of incarcerated parents and was intended to provide parents with motivation, knowledge, and skills relevant to their role in the prevention of the development of antisocial behavior and associated problem behaviors in their children. In prior analyses of data drawn from the study of focus here, PIO was found to have positive main effects in a number of areas, including arrests (Eddy, Martinez, & Burraston, 2013; Eddy, Martinez, Burraston, & Newton, 2016), and thus moderation analyses are warranted. Here, we examine the potential influence of one theoretically based moderator, living with children before incarceration.

A theory-based moderator: Living with children

Based on Hirschi's social attachment theory and Laub and Sampson's life-course paradigm, living with one's child before incarceration and the PIO intervention should be protective factors in reducing recidivism. Living with a child before incarceration presumably would facilitate greater involvement between parent and child and foster stronger parent–child attachments. Similarly, the PIO intervention should increase parent–child attachments, commitment, and involvement by teaching parenting skills and motivating parents to use their new knowledge and skills to be a better parent. In recidivism research, the effects of a treatment are typically found to be strongest among the highest-risk cases compared with lower-risk cases (see Gaes, Flanagan, Motiuk, & Stewart, 1999). Here, those at greater "risk" would be parents who did not live with their children before being incarcerated. We expect that these parents should benefit more from the PIO intervention than those who had lived with their child previously.

Hypotheses

We hypothesize that living with a child before incarceration will moderate the effect of the PIO intervention on outcomes. Specifically, the impact of the intervention on parents who did not live with their child before incarceration will be greater than that on parents who did live with their child previously. However, PIO will benefit participants who did and who did not live with their child before incarceration.

Method

Study design

The Parent Child Study was a randomized controlled trial that compared outcomes for incarcerated fathers and mothers assigned to the PIO or the control condition. The study was conducted in close collaboration with the Oregon Department of Corrections (DOC) and Pathfinders of Oregon, a nonprofit service delivery agency with extensive experience working in the DOC. Incarcerated parents were recruited from all 14 state correctional facilities in Oregon. However, for the study, the PIO intervention was conducted only within four of the "releasing institutions" where inmates serve the final portions of their sentence before release. Three of the four releasing institutions were for men and one was for women; each ranged from minimum to medium security. Inmates who expressed interest in participating in the program and met the eligibility criteria were transferred to one of the four institutions if they did not already reside in one of them. To ensure a demographically diverse sample, women and minorities were oversampled from the eligible pool. After recruitment, participants were randomly assigned into conditions and then assessed before the start of the PIO intervention, following the intervention, 6 months after release, and 1 year after release. The study was approved by the federal Office of Human Research Protections and overseen by the Oregon Social Learning Center Institutional Review Board.

The seven eligibility criteria for study participants were (a) at least one minor child (target age from 3 to 11 years), (b) the legal right to contact the child, (c) some role in parenting the child in the past and an expectation of playing some role in the future, (d) had contact information for the caregiver of the child, (e) did not commit a crime against a child or a sex offense, (f) less than 9 months left from the end of his/her prison sentence, and (g) the DOC was willing to transfer him or her to one of the four study institutions. Recruitment involved advertisements in inmate newspapers, posters on bulletin boards, announcements during inmate club meetings, and special meetings about parenting. There were 453 inmates who expressed interest in participating in the program and met the eligibility criteria; of those, 359 (about 80%) consented to participate in the study. The overall participation rate for fathers and mothers was high; however, the participation rate for mothers (92%) was significantly ($p < .05$) higher than for fathers (68%). The majority of men who chose not to participate did so because they did not want to transfer to a different facility (i.e., 51 of 77). Randomization into condition was at the individual level, blocking on sex, race, and ethnicity. Randomization occurred within institution-based cohorts before the start of each new PIO session. Further details on the study design are provided in Eddy, Martinez, and Burraston (2013).

Sample

Of the 359 participants, 161 (45%) were men and 198 (55%) were women. In terms of race and ethnicity, 59% of the participants were White, 13% were African American, 11% were multiracial, 8% were Native American, and 8% were Latino. In terms of education, 37% of the participants had less than a high school education, 31% had a high school diploma or GED, and 32% had at least some post–high school training or college (less than 1% had a college degree). Parents, on average, had three children, most of whom were biological. In the month before incarceration, 34% of the parents had lived with their child full-time, and 9% had lived with them part-time. About 25% of parents had no contact with their child during the month before incarceration. None of these values differed significantly by gender. Men were more likely to be sentenced for a crime against a person (61% versus 40%, $p < .001$), to be serving a longer sentence than women (2.2 years versus 1.5 years, $p < .001$), and to have been in the custody of DOC more frequently (1.7 times versus 1.4 times, $p < .001$). Approximately 93% of women and 87% of men had a history of drug and/or alcohol abuse or addiction ($p < .05$). There were also significant gender differences on mental health problems (27% of men and 47% of women, $p < .001$). Participants in the intervention and control conditions did not differ significantly on any of these factors.

Conditions

The PIO intervention was delivered within a group-based format with approximately 15 participants per group. Groups met for 2.5-hour sessions, 3 times per week, across 12 weeks, for a total time of 90 hours of instruction. In addition to the content and activities noted here, PIO includes instruction on communication and cooperation with the child's caregiver and other adults, thoughtful decision making around romantic partners after release, child development, child health and safety, and positive parenting from prison. PIO also includes individual meetings between the parent and instructor to discuss unique family circumstances and to determine if referrals for other services are needed.

The control group received "services-as-usual," which was whatever parenting program the releasing institution normally provided. Most institutions did not provide such a service at the time of this study or, if they did, not many parents received it. If there was a service available, it was typically lecture based and focused on how participants were parented and provided little, if any, time for the practice of parenting skills. Participants in the control condition were not eligible to enroll in the PIO class, but they were eligible for all other programs and services for which they qualified based on DOC requirements.

Assessments

There was a wide variety of literacy levels among the participants; therefore, all interviews were conducted verbally. Participants were compensated for their time for each interview (on average, $30 per interview). Table 1 contains descriptive statistics by condition for the variables used in the model and described here later.

Dependent variable

Postrelease arrests

The dependent variable is the total number of arrests in the first year after the release from prison. Postrelease arrests were extracted from official police records for the 359 participants.

Independent variables

Condition

The independent variable of most interest is condition, which is a dummy variable code "1" if the subjects were in the PIO condition and "0" if they were in the control condition.

Table 1. Descriptive Statistics.

	PIO Intervention		Control	
Variable	Mean (Count)	SD (Count)	Mean (Count)	SD (Count)
Dependent variable				
Postrelease arrests	1.35	3.77	1.41	4.01
Independent variables				
Intervention	(195)		(165)	
Lived with child	(90 no)	(104 yes)		
Control variables				
Gender	(107 men)	(87 women)	(91 men)	(74 women)
Prior arrests	17.21	13.44	16.61	12.37
Years incarcerated	1.46	1.68	1.36	1.49
Years incarcerated (log transformed)	−0.06	0.90	−0.09	0.87
Family contact	4.67	7.55	5.01	8.34
Family contact (log transformed)	1.09	1.10	1.14	1.08
Mental health diagnoses	0.08	0.32	0.08	0.40
Age	31.20	6.71	31.67	6.60

Lived with child
The variable "parent lived with child before incarceration" is from the preintervention interview with the incarcerated parent. It is a dichotomous dummy variable coded "0" if the parent did not live with the child in the month before incarceration and coded "1" if the parent did live with the child at any time during that month (even if it was only part of the month).

Interaction: Condition × Lived with child
The interaction variable (moderator) is the product of the variables condition and lived with child (condition × lived with child). Including the interaction in the model with condition and lived with child allows the relationship between lived with child and the dependent variable "postrelease arrests" to vary by condition.

Control variables

Prior arrests
Prior arrests are the total arrests before the current incarceration. It is based on official police records for 345 participants. No arrest records were collected for the 14 participants who refused to provide consent for the records search. Of the 14 missing cases, 3 are from the control group and 11 are from the treatment group.

Time in prison
Time in prison is the total number of years the parent had been continuously incarcerated before the start of the intervention. This sum was provided by the DOC. Total time in prison was highly skewed; therefore, it was natural log transformed to normalize its distribution.

Age
Age is the age of the participant in years. Age is included in the model because it is common for people to commit fewer crimes as they become older.

Gender
Women are coded "1" and men are coded "0."

Mental health and/or learning diagnoses
This variable is the total number of mental health and/or learning problems diagnosed by the DOC before the start of the intervention. It was provided by the DOC.

Family contact

Family contact in prison is the total number of in person, phone, and letter contacts by family members during the month before the preintervention interview and was provided by the incarcerated parent. It has an extremely skewed distribution, so we normalized its distribution by log transforming it (i.e., 1 plus the natural log of total family contact).

Analytic strategy

STATA 13 Zero-Inflated Negative Binomial Regression (ZINB) was used to test the hypothesized interaction. ZINB allowed for the control of the over-inflation of zeros in the count of postrelease arrests and for overdispersion (Cameron & Trivedi, 1998; Rabe-Hesketh Skrondal, 2012). In addition, adjusted standard errors were used to correct for nesting by prisons.

Two ZINB models were tested. Model 1 contained condition, lived with child, and the control variables gender, total arrests before incarceration, total years incarcerated (log transformed), family contact, and learning and mental health diagnoses. Model 2 contained all the variables from Model 1 plus the interaction variable (condition × lived with child). To test the moderating hypothesis, that the effect of lived with child prior to incarceration on postrelease arrests varies by condition (PIO versus control), we included the variables condition, lived with child, and the interaction variable (condition × lived with child).

There were 22 missing cases on the variable on family contact at the preintervention assessment point and 14 cases missing prior arrests. A "best practice" in handling missing data was used, namely multiple imputation (Boldner, 2008; Collins, Schafer, & Kam, 2001; Graham, Cumsille, & Elek-Fisk, 2003; Johnson & Young, 2011). We used the multiple imputation procedure in STATA statistical software (Stata Corp, 2013) to impute missing cases. For each missing value, we imputed 50 values and then used the mean of these values as the final imputed value (Boldner, 2008). The imputation of data did not change any of the results. Intervention participants were included in analyses regardless of whether they attended PIO sessions (i.e., an "intent-to-treat" approach appropriate to a randomized controlled trial was used).

Results

Model 1

In Model 1, the condition dummy variable was significant (incident rate ratio [IRR] = .586, $p < .01$). The PIO intervention group had 41.4% fewer arrests than the control group, controlling for the variables in the model (see Table 2). We only report the condition dummy variable in Model 1 because the interaction variable (condition × lived with child) in Model 2 was significant.

Model 2

The ZINB regression coefficients, IRRs, and significance levels for Model 2 are listed in Table 2. While our focus in this study was the interaction between the intervention dummy variable and lived with child, it is worth noting that all of the variables in the negative binomial portion of the model except for age and family contact were significant, and all but the condition dummy variable in the zero inflation portion of the model were significant. In Model 2, all of the variables combined to explain 22% of the variation in postrelease arrests. The condition dummy variable (IRR = 0.46, $p < .01$), lived with child (IRR = 0.63, $p < .001$), and their interaction (IRR = 1.65, $p < .05$) were all significant. The significant interaction means the magnitude of the PIO treatment on postrelease arrests varied based on whether the parent lived with their child before incarceration.

Figure 1 is the predicted number of total postrelease arrests by condition and parent lived with child before incarceration, plotted for males at mean levels of the control variables. As hypothesized, participants in the control condition who did not live with their child before incarceration had the highest level of postrelease arrests followed by participants in the control condition who lived with their child before incarceration. Living with child before incarceration is only significant for the control condition, while there

Table 2. Zero Inflated Negative Binomial Regression Model Predicting Total Postrelease Arrests.

	IRR	Coefficient	95% CI
Total postrelease arrests			
Condition	0.46	−0.77**	−1.26, −0.29
Lived with child	0.63	−0.47***	−0.70, −0.24
Interaction (condition × lived with child)	1.65	0.50*	0.01, 0.99
Prior arrests	1.03	0.03**	0.01, 0.05
Female	0.48	−0.74***	−0.94, −0.53
Years incarcerated (log transformed)	1.54	0.43***	0.25, 0.62
Family contact (log transformed)	0.99	−0.01	−0.18, 0.16
Age	0.99	−0.01	−0.03, 0.01
Mental health diagnoses	0.13	−2.04***	−2.65, −1.44
Constant	—	1.61***	0.81, 2.41
Inflation			
Condition		−0.34	−0.84, 0.16
Prior arrests		−0.04***	−0.07, −0.02
Mental health diagnoses		−13.97***	−15.78, −12.17
Constant		1.32***	0.75, 1.90
Ln(α)		−0.29	−1.02, 0.44
α		0.75	0.36, 1.55
Maximum likelihood R^2		0.22	

Note. *$p < .05$; **$p < .01$; ***$p < .001$.

[Bar chart showing Total Post Release Arrests by four groups: Control: Did Not Live with Child Prior (~2.0), Control: Lived with Child Prior (~1.25), PIO: Did Not Live with Child Prior (~1.1), PIO: Lived with Child Prior (~1.15).]

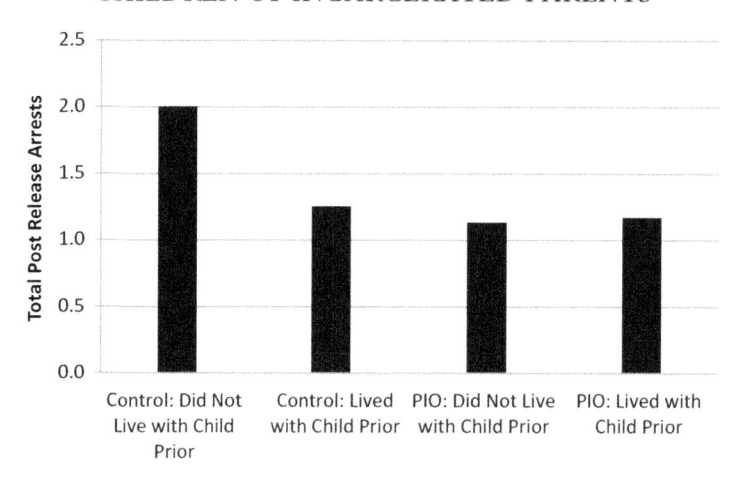

Figure 1. Interaction between condition and lived with child before incarceration predicting total postrelease arrests for men at mean level of control variables.

is little difference in postrelease arrests for the PIO group regardless of whether or not a participant lived with their child before incarceration.

Of note is that there was virtually no difference between the participants in the PIO condition who lived with their child before incarceration and those in the PIO condition who did not. In addition, participants in both of these subgroups had significant fewer rearrests than participants in the control group who did not live with their child before incarceration. Although participants in both of PIO subgroups had fewer postrelease arrests than participants in the control condition whose parents lived with their child before incarceration, the difference was minimal and not significant. For women, Figure 1 would look identical except with 52% fewer arrests in each category (IRR = .48, $p < .001$).

For each additional prior arrest, the IRR for postrelease arrests increased 1.03 times ($p < .01$), while holding all other variables in the model constant. For each unit increase in years in prison (log transformed), the IRR increased 1.54 times ($p < .001$). The relationship between mental health and/or learning diagnoses with postrelease rearrests was more complicated than the other control variables, because the relationship in the negative binomial model was in the opposite direction as that of the zero inflation model. Those with mental health and/or learning diagnoses were more likely to get rearrested (based on the zero inflation model) but were less likely to be rearrested multiple times (based on the negative binomial portion of the model).

Total prior arrests and mental health and/or learning diagnoses both significantly predicted the zero inflation. While condition was not related to the zero inflation ($p > .05$), total prior arrests was negatively related to the zero inflation ($b = -0.04$; $p < .001$). Similarly, mental health and or learning diagnoses were negatively related to the zero inflation ($b = -13.94$; $p = .000$).

Discussion

The PIO program shows promise as one component in a preventive intervention strategy designed to ease a person's reentry into society and prevent recidivism. In these analyses, overall, participants in the PIO intervention condition had 41.4% fewer arrests after release than participants in the services as usual control group. Given that participants were randomized to condition, this is strong preliminary evidence that the PIO intervention played some role as a turning point for those who lived with their child before incarceration and for those who did not. Such a finding is in need of replication.

Beyond this, however, the interaction between intervention condition (PIO versus control) and lived with child before incarceration was also significant. Participants in the control condition who lived with their child before incarceration had 37.4% fewer arrests than participants in the control condition who did not live with their child before incarceration. Thus, for participants in the control condition, incarceration per se seems to have acted as a turning point for those who lived with their child before incarceration, but not for those who did not live with their child previously. As hypothesized, this may be due to those who lived with their child before incarceration having a stronger parent–child bond (attachment) and parent–caregiver bonds and/or such individuals simply may have had more family support after release.

In contrast, in the PIO condition, the intervention appears to have worked as a turning point for those who lived with their child before incarceration and for those who did not live with their child before incarceration. Participants in the PIO condition who lived with their child before incarceration had 52.2% fewer arrests than participants in the control condition who did not live with their child before incarceration and, although not significant, 23.7% fewer arrests than participants in the control group who lived with their child before incarceration. Similarly, participants in the PIO condition who did not live with their child before incarceration had 53.6% fewer arrests than participants in the control condition who did not live with their child before incarceration and, again, although not significant, 26.3% fewer arrests than the control group who lived with their child before incarceration. There were virtually no differences in postrelease arrests between participants in the PIO condition who lived with their child before incarceration and participants in the PIO condition who did not live with their child previously.

The success of participants in the PIO condition, regardless of their living situation before incarceration, may be due to an increase in parent–child bonds (attachment), parent–parent attachment, and/or family social support. Eddy et al. (2013) provide evidence of this is in their findings of significant improvements for participants in the PIO condition in terms of parent–child positive interaction, improvement in their relationship with the primary caregiver of their child, and increasing the likelihood they thought they would play an active role in their child's life.

Future research should examine other possible theoretically based mediators between PMT interventions with incarcerated parents and postrelease arrests and other important outcomes of interest. Considering these findings altogether, there is evidence that a PMT intervention acted as a significant turning point toward desisting from crime. Additional studies, particularly randomized controlled trials, are needed of PMT interventions to replicate and extend these findings.

Based on the findings here, PIO shows initial promise as one component in a preventive intervention strategy targeting the reentry period. In our opinion, the potential power of psychosocial interventions alone, even cognitive-behavioral evidence-based programs, to address recidivism should not be overestimated. There are many other issues beyond family bonds and relationship support that can lead to poor outcomes during the reentry period, and ignoring these in reentry programs is problematic. Clear challenges that must be faced but that can be incredibly difficult to overcome and can have a powerful impact on success on the outside include securing housing, finding a job, avoiding association with criminal associates, and addressing mental and physical health needs and substance abuse problems. PMT seems best thought of as an adjunct to a multimodal intervention that takes a holistic approach to the prevention of recidivism.

Funding

This study was supported by Grants MH46690 and MH6553 from the Division of Epidemiology and Services Research, National Institute of Mental Health (NIMH), National Institutes of Health (NIH), U.S. PHS; by Grant HD054480 from the Social and Affective Development/Child Maltreatment and Violence, National Institute of Child Health and Human Development, NIH, U.S. PHS; by a grant from the Edna McConnell Clark Foundation; and through funding from the legislature of the state of Oregon.

References

Bales, W. D., & Mears, D. P. (2008). Inmate social ties and the transition to society: Does visitation reduce recidivism? *Journal of Research in Crime and Delinquency, 45,* 287–321. doi:10.1177/0022427808317574

Bodner, T. (2008). What improves with increased missing data imputations? *Structural Equation Modeling: A Multidisciplinary Journal, 15,* 651–675. doi:10.1080/10705510802339072

Braman, D. S. (2004). *Doing time on the outside: Incarceration and family life in urban America.* Ann Arbor, MI: University of Michigan Press.

Brestan, E. V., & Eyberg, S. M. (1998). Effective psychosocial treatments of conduct-disordered children and adolescents: 29 years, 82 studies, and 5,272 kids. *Journal of Clinical Child Psychology, 27,* 180–189.

Cairns, R. B., & Cairns, B. D. (1994). *Lifelines and risks.* New York, NY: Cambridge University Press.

Cameron, A. C., & Trivedi, P. (1998). *Regression analysis of count data.* New York, NY: Cambridge University Press.

Carson, E. A. (2015). *Prisoners in 2014.* NCJ 248955. Washington, DC: U.S. Department of Justice, Bureau of Justice Statistics. Retrieved from http://www.bjs.gov/content/pub/pdf/p14.pdf

Caspi, A., & Elder, G. H. (1988). Childhood precursors of the life course: Early personality and life disorganization. In E. M. Hetherington, R. M. Lerner, & M. Perlmutter (Eds.), *Child development in life-span perspective* (pp. 115–142). Hillsdale, NJ: Erlbaum.

Collins, L. M., Schafer, J. L., & Kam, C. M. (2001). A comparison of inclusive and restrictive strategies in modern missing data procedures. *Psychological Methods, 6*(4), 330–351. doi:10.1037/1082-989X.6.4.330

Durose, M. R., Cooper, A. D., & Snyder, H. N. (2014). *Recidivism of prisoners released in 30 states in 2005: Patterns from 2005 to 2010* NCJ 244205. Washington, DC: U.S. Department of Justice, Bureau of Justice Statistics.

Eddy, J. M., Kjellstrand, J., Martinez, C. R., Jr., & Newton, R. (2010). Theory-based multimodal parenting intervention for incarcerated parents and their children. In J. M. Eddy, & J. Poehlmann (Eds.), *Children of incarcerated parents: A handbook for researchers and practitioners* (pp. 237–264). Washington, DC: The Urban Institute Press.

Eddy, J. M., Martinez, C. R., Jr., & Burraston, B. (2013). A randomized control trial of parent management training program for incarcerated parents: Proximal impacts. *Monographs of the Society for Research in Child Development 78(3):* 75–93.

Eddy, J. M., Martinez, C. R., Jr., Burraston, B., & Newton, R. (2016). *A randomized control trial of parent management training program for incarcerated parents: Distal impacts.* Manuscript submitted for publication.

Eddy, J. M., Martinez, C. R., Jr., Schiffmann, T., Newton, R., Olin, L., Leve, L. ... Shortt, J. W. (2008). Development of a multisystemic parent management training intervention for incarcerated parents, their children and families. *Clinical Psychologist, 12*(3), 86–98. doi:10.1080/13284200802495461

Edin, K., Nelson, T. J., & Paranal, R. (2004). Fatherhood and incarceration as potential turning points in the criminal careers of unskilled men. In M. Pattillo, D. Weiman, & B. Western (Eds), *Imprisoning America: The social effects of mass incarceration* (pp. 46–75). New York, NY: Russell Sage Foundation.

Forgatch, M. S., & Martinez, C. R., Jr. (1999). Parent management training: A program linking basic research and practical application. *Journal of the Norwegian Psychological Society, 36*, 923–937.

Foster, H., & Hagan, J. (2007). Incarceration and intergenerational social exclusion. *Social Problems, 54*(4), 399–433. doi:10.1525/sp.2007.54.4.399

Gaes, G., Flanagan, T., Motiuk, L., & Stewart, L. (1999). Adult correctional treatment. *Crime and Justice, 26*, 361–426. doi:10.1086/449300

Geller, A., Garfinkel, I., & Western, B. (2011). Paternal incarceration and support for children in fragile families. *Demography, 48*, 25–47. doi:10.1007/s13524-010-0009-9

Geller, A., & Walker Franklin, A. (2014). Paternal incarceration and the housing security of urban mothers. *Journal of Marriage and Family, 76*, 411–427. doi:10.1111/jomf.2014.76.issue-2

Gendreau, P., Little, T., & Goggin, C. (1996). A meta-analysis of the predictors of adult offender recidivism: What works! *Criminology, 34*, 575–607. doi:10.1111/j.1745-9125.1996.tb01220.x

Glaze, L. E., & Maruschak, L. M. (2010). *Parents in prison and their minor children* NCJ 222984. Washington, DC: U.S. Department of Justice, Bureau of Justice Statistics.

Graham, J., Cumsille, P., & Elek-Fisk, E. (2003). Methods for handling missing data. In J. Graham (Eds.), *Handbook of psychology* (Vol. 2, pp. 87–114). Hoboken, NJ: Wiley.

Grinstead, O., Faigeles, B., Bancroft, C., & Zack, B. (2001). The financial cost of maintaining relationships with incarcerated African American men: A survey of women prison visitors. *Journal of African American Men, 6*(1), 59–69. doi:10.1007/s12111-001-1014-2

Hetherington, E. M., & Baltes, P. B. (1988). Child psychology and life-span development. In E. M. Hetherington, & R. M. Lerner (Eds.), *Child development in life-span perspective* (pp. 1–19). Hillsdale, NJ: Lawrence Erlbaum Associates.

Hirschi, T. (2002). *Causes of delinquency*. New Brunswick, NJ: Transaction Publishers. (Original work published 1969)

Hughes, M. (1998). Turning points in the lives of young inner-city men forgoing destructive criminal behaviors: A qualitative study. *Social Work Research, 22*(3), 143–151. doi:10.1033/swr/22.3.143

Johnson, D. R., & Young, R. (2011). Towards best practices in analyzing datasets with missing data: Comparisons and recommendations. *Journal of Marriage and Family, 73*, 926–945. doi:10.1111/j.1741-3737.2011.00861.x

Langan, P. A., & Levin, D. J. (2002). Recidivism of prisoners released in 1994. *Federal Sentencing Reporter, 15*(1), 58–65. doi:10.1525/fsr.2002.15.1.58

Laub, J. H., & Sampson, R. J. (2001). Understanding desistance from crime. *Crime and Justice, 28*, 1–69. Retrieved from http://www.jstor.org/stable/1147672

Lopoo, L. M., & Western, B. (2005). Incarceration and the formation and stability of marital unions. *Journal of Marriage and Family, 67*(3), 721–734. doi:10.1111/jomf.2005.67.issue-3

Magnusson, D., & Torestad, B. (1993). A holistic view of personality: A model revisited. *Annual Review of Psychology, 44*, 427–452. doi:10.1146/annurev.psych.44.1.427

Maruschak, L. M., Glaze, L. E., & Mumola, C. J. (2010). Incarcerated parents and their children. In J. M. Eddy & J. Poehlmann (Eds.), *Children of incarcerated parents: A handbook for researchers and practitioners* (pp. 33–51). Washington, DC: Urban Institute Press.

Mumola, C. J. (2000). *Incarcerated parents and their children.* Washington, DC: U.S. Department of Justice. Retrieved from http://www.ojp.usdoj.gov/bjs/pub/pdf/iptc.pdf

Murphey, D., & Cooper, P. M. (2015). *Parents behind bars: What happens to their children?* Bethesda, MD: Child Trends, Childtrends.org. Retrieved from http://www.childtrends.org/wp-content/uploads/2015/10/2015-42ParentsBehindBars.pdf

Ndrecka, M. (2014). *The impact of reentry programs on recidivism: A meta-analysis.* (Electronic thesis or dissertation). Retrieved from https://etd.ohiolink.edu/

Nelson, M., Deess, P., & Allen, C. (1999). *The first month out: Post-incarceration experiences in New York City.* New York, NY: Vera Institute of Justice.

Patterson, G. R. (1982). Observations of family process. In G. R. Patterson (Ed.), *Coercive family process: A social learning approach* (Vol. 3, pp. 41–65). Eugene, OR: Castalia.

Patterson, G. R., Capaldi, D. C., & Bank, L. (1991). An early starter model for predicting delinquency. In D. J. Pepler, & K. H. Rubin (Eds.), *The development and treatment of childhood aggression.* Hillsdale, NJ: Erlbaum.

Patterson, G. R., Reid, J. B., & Dishion, T. J. (1992). *A social learning approach: Antisocial boys* (Vol. IV). Eugene, OR: Castalia.

Rabe-Hesketh, S., & Skrondal, A. (2012). *Multilevel and longitudinal modeling using stata: Categorical responses, counts, and survival* (3rd ed., Vol. II). College Station, TX: Stata Press.

Reid, J. B., & Eddy, J. M. (1997). The prevention of antisocial behavior: Some considerations in the search for effective interventions. In D. M. Stoff, J. Breiling, & J. D. Maser (Eds.), *Handbook of antisocial behavior* (pp. 343–356). New York, NY: Wiley.

Reid, J. B., Patterson, G. R., & Snyder, J. (Eds.). (2002). *Antisocial behavior in children and adolescents: A developmental analysis and model for intervention.* Washington, DC: American Psychological Association.

Rutter, M. (1989). Pathways from childhood to adult life. *Journal of Child Psychology and Psychiatry, 30*, 23–51. doi:10.1111/j.1469-7610.1989.tb00768.x

Sampson, R. J., & Laub, J. H. (1993). *Crime in the making: Pathways and turning points through life.* Cambridge, MA: Harvard University Press.

Schiffmann, T., Eddy, J. M., Martinez, C. R., Leve, L., & Newton, R. (2008). *Parenting inside out: Parent management training for incarcerated parents in prison.* Portland, OR: Oregon Social Learning Center and Children's Justice Alliance.

Schmidt, P., & White, A. D. (1989). Predicting criminal recidivism using split population survival time models. *Journal of Econometrics, 40*, 141–159. doi:10.1016/0304-4076(89)90034-1

StataCorp. (2013). *Stata multiple-imputation reference manual: Release 13.* [Statistical Software]. College Station, TX: StataCorp LP.

Travis, J. (2000). *But they all come back: Rethinking prisoner reentry.* [Research in Brief]. Washington, DC: National Institute of Justice.

Travis, J., Western, B., & Redburn, S. (Eds.). (2014). *The growth of incarceration in the United States: Exploring causes and consequences.* Washington, DC: National Academies Press.

Turney, K., & Wildeman, C. (2013). Redefining relationships: Explaining the countervailing consequences of paternal incarceration for parenting. *American Sociological Review, 78*(6), 949–979. doi:10.1177/0003122413505589

Webster-Stratton, C., & Taylor, T. (2001). Nipping early risk factors in the bud: Preventing substance abuse, delinquency, and violence in adolescence through interventions targeted at young children (0-8 years). *Prevention Science, 2,* 165–192. doi:10.1023/A:1011510923900

Western, B., & Wildeman, C. (2009). The black family and mass incarceration. *The ANNALS of the American Academy of Political and Social Science, 621,* 221–242. doi:10.1177/0002716208324850

Wildeman, C. (2014). Parental incarceration, child homelessness, and the invisible consequences of mass imprisonment. *The ANNALS of the American Academy of Political and Social Science, 651*(1), 74–96. doi:10.1177/0002716213502921

Building a Tailored, Multilevel Prevention Strategy to Support Children and Families Affected by Parental Incarceration

Jean Kjellstrand, PhD

ABSTRACT
During the past several decades, a wave of incarceration engulfed the United States. In the wake of this "mass incarceration" are children and families who continue to struggle from its impact. Although findings are now emerging on the impacts of incarceration, there are few studies that have examined how to best intervene to promote positive development for those children who have had a parent incarcerated. While there are common risks and challenges faced by children and their families, the significant variation between and among these individuals and their relationships highlights the challenges in finding solutions. Given the number of issues at play, it is clear that a "one-size-fits-all" approach to addressing child needs is not sufficient. This article examines some of the common challenges faced by families impacted by parental incarceration as well as existing interventions designed to help support children and families overcome these challenges. It then offers some potential directions for the field to move, to develop a prevention strategy that meets the needs within the population and leads to better outcomes for the children of incarcerated parents, their families, and their communities.

Between 1970 and 2000, a wave of incarceration engulfed the United States. The number of adults incarcerated in state and federal prisons increased five-fold, from 320,000 to nearly 1.4 million (Maruschak & Mumola, 2010). The increase was, at least in part, a result of three intersecting dynamics. The first was a shift in policymakers' view of the role and goals of the criminal justice system, which changed from one of rehabilitation to one of retribution; the second was the politicization of responses to crime, which decreased judicial influence on sentencing and led to such practices as mandatory and extended sentencing for drug and other offenses; the third was the commercialization of prisons, whereby prisons became a business venture, particularly for financially stressed rural communities (Pizzarro, Stenius, & Pratt, 2006).

In the wake of this "mass incarceration" are children and families who continue to struggle from its impact. By 2007, more than 1.7 million minor children had at least one parent in prison (Maruschak & Mumola, 2010). The number of children who had experienced parental incarceration over their lifetime was nearly five times this amount (Kjellstrand & Eddy, 2011; Western & Wildeman, 2009). Research indicates that the effects of parental incarceration are varied and complex. Arrest and incarceration of a parent are not typically the start of problems for a child and family, but rather new episodes in an already difficult life situation that is often marked not only by family challenges, such as poverty, an unstable home life, and parental substance abuse and other mental health problems but also by community-level challenges, such as neighborhood socioeconomic disadvantage, community disorganization, and violent crime (Johnston, 1995; Nichols & Loper, 2012; Travis, Waul, & Geraghty, 2004).

Developmental research during the past 20 years has established that exposure to any of the aforementioned risks increases the likelihood of problematic outcomes for children including delinquency, depression, and substance abuse (Ackerman, Brown, & Izard, 2004; Connell & Goodman, 2002; Lipsey & Derzon, 1998). The children of incarcerated parents are often exposed to several of these risks at once. An individual risk factor can be detrimental to the development of a child, but the combined effect of multiple risks and the subsequent transaction between and among risks over time can be especially toxic (Gutman, Sameroff, & Cole, 2003; Masten & Coatsworth, 1998; Wachs, 1996).

While findings continue to emerge on the effects that parental incarceration can have on children and families, there are few studies that have examined how best to intervene to promote positive development for those children who have, or have had, a parent incarcerated. Researchers have identified many of the common risks and challenges faced by children, their incarcerated parents, and their families (Eddy & Poehlmann, 2010). However, the variation between and among families highlights the challenge in finding solutions. The degree that parental incarceration affects a child depends on the strengths and needs of the child, their family, and their community, as well as aspects specific to the incarceration history, such as parent functioning before and during incarceration, the timing and length of incarceration, the nature of parent–child contact during incarceration, and the level of disruption of caregiving relationships and family circumstances due to incarceration (Arditti, 2012; Cho, 2010; Foster, 2011; Turanovic, Rodriguez, & Pratt, 2012).

Given the number of issues at play, it is clear that a "one-size-fits-all" approach to addressing child and family needs is not sufficient. Rather, intervention strategies are needed that both address common challenges facing families with an incarcerated parent, yet are flexible enough to accommodate specific child and family differences. At the same time, strategies are needed for reducing harmful influences and building protective elements within the communities in which the children of incarcerated parents are living.

These ideas were supported in a recent National Research Council and Institute of Medicine report (2009) that stressed the importance of multi-component and multilevel (i.e., child, family, and communities) approaches to promote positive development among children. In working with children of incarcerated parents, this will likely be especially important given the number of risks that frequently come into play. This article examines some of the existing interventions designed to address common challenges faced by families impacted by parental incarceration as well as to promote positive outcomes. It then offers some potential directions for the field to move to develop a prevention strategy to meet the needs of the population and that results in better outcomes for not only for the children of incarcerated parents and their families but for their communities as well.

Existing interventions to assist children and families with an incarcerated parent

What follows is a brief summary of some of the more commonly discussed interventions that are intended to address the risks facing children of incarcerated parents. For convenience, the interventions have been grouped into three general categories: parent/family support, child adjustment, and the broader family/community context. When such exists, efficacy information about the interventions is included. Unfortunately, very few of these interventions have been rigorously tested using samples of children of incarcerated parents and their families.

Parent/family support

Parent and family intervention programs are often advocated to mitigate risk within criminal justice–involved families (e.g., Eddy, Kjellstrand, Martinez, & Newton, 2010). By helping to improve communication and interpersonal relationships within families, such programs are seen as a way to promote positive child development and encourage family support after release but also decrease the likelihood of recidivism of the formerly incarcerated parent (Bales & Mears, 2008; Baumer, O'Donnell, & Hughes, 2009; La Vigne, Naser, Brooks, & Castro, 2005; Reid, Patterson, & Snyder, 2002). Family-focused programs may take multiple forms, including parenting classes, visitation, and alternative living situations and may be offered by a variety of entities (e.g., prisons, social services, nonprofit agencies).

Parenting classes

By developing positive parenting skills, parenting classes are believed to increase the likelihood of prosocial child development for children of incarcerated parents and decrease the likelihood that these children will enter the criminal justice system (Loper & Novero, 2010). This perception is based on the wealth of research demonstrating the relationship between the heightened risk for antisocial behavior and poor parenting and the benefit of parenting programs (Reid, Patterson, & Snyder, 2002). Recent research on parenting intervention programs for criminal justice–involved parents, albeit limited, has found some similar benefits. Specifically, programs have been shown to result in an increase in parenting proficiency, parenting knowledge, self-esteem, improved parent–child and parent–home caregiver interactions, and a reduction in parenting stress and depression (Eddy, Martinez, & Burraston, 2013; Gonzalez, Romero, & Cerbana, 2007; Loper & Tuerk, 2011). While the programs vary considerably in terms of objectives, length, and delivery, the typical curriculum offers information on effective parenting skills and child development with a goal of improving parenting and outcomes for children (e.g., Parenting Inside Out: Eddy, Martinez, Schiffmann, Newton, Olin, Leve, & Shortt, 2008; Partners in Parenting: Gonzalez, Romero, & Cerbano, 2007; Parenting from Inside: Loper & Tuerk, 2011; Parenting While Incarcerated: Miller et al., 2014). Some countries have established parenting classes for nonincarcerated caregivers; however, within the United States, parenting classes most often target incarcerated or formerly incarcerated parents only (Parke & Clarke-Stewart, 2001).

Visitation and remote contact

An increasing number of correctional institutions offer specialized visitation programs for inmate parents and their children (e.g., Family Ties through the Osborne Association in NYC; Girl Scouts Beyond Bars in several cities throughout the United States). These programs vary in the nature and may incorporate such visitation enhancements as a "child-friendly" room for children and parents, flexible visiting hours, transportation to and from the institution, and special events for families (Clement, 1993). Typically, program goals focus on minimizing the separation of a parent and child and maintaining and/or strengthening the parent–child relationship. While research on visitation programs per se is sparse, in general, research has found parent–child visits beneficial for incarcerated parents. However, results are mixed in terms of the benefits to children. Most notably, the benefits of the visits appear to be the greatest for the children when the visitation program is part of a larger intervention program for families (Poehlmann, Dallaire, Loper, & Shear, 2010). Remote contact (e.g., letters, phone calls, televisitation) provides additional ways for parents and children to connect with one another (Poehlmann et al., 2010). While research is minimal around the benefits of these different methods of contact, initial findings suggest that such alternative forms of contact are beneficial to the incarcerated parent (i.e., diminished stress, increased sense of parenting competency) and child (i.e., reduced depression, somatic complaints, and feelings of alienation).

Prison nurseries

Once widespread but currently rare within the United States, prison nurseries (e.g., at Bedford Hills Correctional Facility in New York State; at the Washington State Corrections Center for Women) offer a way for incarcerated mothers to raise their infants during incarceration. Generally, these programs house mothers and their children in special wings of a facility and limit the age of the infant who can live in a nursery from birth to 12–18 months (Parke & Clarke-Stewart, 2001). The basic assumption with these programs is that keeping an infant and a mother together during this early stage of development helps increase mother–child bonding, which, in turn, improves child adjustment. While little rigorous research has been done on these programs, initial findings indicate that prison nurseries and supplemental parenting guidance help facilitate mother–child attachment and improve maternal parenting (Byrne, Goshin, & Joestl, 2010). Infants appear to be more likely to develop a secure attachment when they reside with their mothers; however, they often experience temporary distress when they are transferred to new caretakers after they "age out" of the program.

Alternatives to incarceration

Community-based sentencing is becoming an increasingly popular and potentially cost-effective option for parents whose offense was minor and/or nonviolent (Parke & Clarke-Stewart, 2001). These include such options as house arrest, halfway houses for mothers and children, substance abuse treatment, and day programs where parents attend a program at the correctional institution during the day but reside in their homes. By allowing parents to remain at home while addressing underlying issues related to their criminality (e.g., substance abuse, poverty, mental illness), specific parent and family risks can be addressed while avoiding potential negative effects related to parental incarceration (e.g., family disruption, diminished financial resources, weakening of parent–child bond, stigma). However, scant research exists on the efficacy of these types of programs, and what research there is rarely examines how these programs affect parenting, family functioning, or child outcomes (Phillips, Gleeson, & Waites-Garrett, 2009; Sevigny, Fuleihan, & Ferdik, 2013).

Child adjustment

A complement to programs with incarcerated parents are programs that work directly with children (Parke & Clarke-Stewart, 2001). The underlying assumption of most children's programs is that parental incarceration is not a normative situation and might be harmful to children. As such, children need help dealing with the problems that can arise due to parental incarceration (Hairston, 2007). These programs vary in format (e.g., one-on-one counseling, group sessions) as well as delivery setting (e.g., clinic, school, social services, prisons). By intervening directly with children, the programs strive to boost children's resiliency by providing them with support around difficult situations or emotions (e.g., stigma of having an incarcerated parent, stress, feelings of isolation) and helping them develop healthy coping and problem-solving skills.

Work with individual children

One of the most commonly advocated programs for children of incarcerated parents is mentoring (e.g., Big Brothers/Big Sisters, Amachi Program), a type of intervention that has increased dramatically during the past several decades (Eddy, Cearley, Bergen, & Stern-Carusone, 2013; Zwiebach, Rhodes, & Dun Rappaport, 2010). Although studies that examine mentoring children of incarcerated parents per se are limited, research on mentoring in general suggests that a long-term relationship with a caring nonparental adult mentor can have a positive impact on a child's resiliency and life outcomes, even in the face of exposure to multiple risks (Rishel, Sales, & Koeske, 2005; Werner, 1989). Mentoring has been shown to increase the likelihood of positive outcomes in many areas such as self-esteem, high school attendance and graduation, relationships, and employment, although most studies have been short term in nature (DuBois, Holloway, Valentine, & Cooper, 2002; Klaw, Rhodes, & Fitzgerald, 2003; Rishel et al., 2005). Mentoring has also been found to decrease the likelihood of behavioral problems including risk taking, violent behavior, substance abuse, and delinquency (Aseltine, Dupre, & Lamlein, 2000; LoSciuto, Rajala, Townsend, & Taylor, 1996), particularly for youth experiencing environmental risks (e.g., within their family and/or community). Preliminary research on mentoring with children of incarcerated parents suggests similar positive effects (Laakso & Nygaard, 2012; Schlafer, Poehlmann, Coffino, & Hanneman, 2009), specifically in the reduction of externalizing and internalizing symptoms as well as an increase in the child's self-confidence, trust, and improved school performance.

Individual therapy (e.g., trauma focused, cognitive-behavioral) and case management are interventions that have also been used with children of incarcerated parents to deal not only with issues related to parental incarceration but also with other compounding risks (Phillips & O'Brien, 2012). Further, there are an increasing number of relevant resources available for providers and the families (e.g., Sesame Street's *Little Children, Big Challenges* Incarceration Toolkit; *Behavioral Toolkit for Providers Working with Children of the Incarcerated and their Families* by the Washington State Department of Social and Health Services). Outcome information on these types of programs and resources is very limited.

Groups

Support groups (e.g., Osborne Association's Rap n'Chat in New York City; Project SEEK in Michigan), youth leadership and/or tutoring programs (e.g., U.S. Dream Academy in Maryland; Hour Children's Teen/Pre-Teen Program in New York), and camps (e.g., Angel Tree Camping in Virginia; Reconciliations' Summer Camps in Nashville, Kids United by Incarceration in Washington State) have also been developed and offered to children of incarcerated parents. In these types of programs, children meet peers who are also experiencing the incarceration of their parent(s) and have the opportunity to talk about their experiences. These programs are believed to help mitigate a sense of shame or stigma associated with having a parent incarcerated and to help promote positive development by addressing issues related to isolation, self-esteem, and challenges that can arise when a parent is incarcerated (Springer, Lynch, & Rubin, 2000; Weissman & LaRue, 1998). Outcomes due to these programs are not well documented.

Broader family/community context

Family context

Four of the most reported challenges faced by incarcerated parents are unemployment, physical and behavioral health problems, inadequate housing, and conflictual relationships (Gaes & Kendig, 2003). Existing interventions targeting these challenges tend not to be specific to incarcerated parents as a subgroup but rather incarcerated individuals in general. The programs are offered either during a sentence, often as release approaches, or after release. A few studies have been conducted on programs focused on employment, mental health (particularly substance abuse treatment), and interpersonal skills and, generally, have suggested positive outcomes (see Eddy et al., 2010).

Not only has research found evidence suggesting the importance of these prerelease and postrelease support to meet the needs of the offenders and their families (Nelson & Trone, 2000), but inmate parents see these services as crucial to their success in reentering the community. For example, as part of the recent Parent Child Study (Eddy et al., 2013), a longitudinal randomized controlled trial examining the effects of the Parenting Inside Out parent management training program, inmate parents who were about to reenter the community were asked what services they felt would be most helpful (before and after release) to better parent their children. The five most identified in-prison services were those that addressed parenting skills, individual and interpersonal skills, contact with family/caregivers, substance abuse/mental health treatment, and employment/education/training, while the five most identified postrelease services included employment, education/training, individual and interpersonal skills, parent skill training, substance abuse/mental health treatment, and contact/relationships with family and caregivers (Eddy, 2014; see Table 1).

While research findings suggest the potential importance of these types of services, access to them varies considerably across correctional institutions and within communities. A recent national survey of the services received by inmate parents (Glaze & Maruschak, 2008) found that approximately one-half of fathers and two-thirds of mothers participated in programs while incarcerated. Mental health programs had the highest rates of participation, with roughly one-third of inmates participating in some type of substance abuse and/or mental health treatment programs. However, only 11% of incarcerated parents who met the criteria for substance abuse treatment actually received residential treatment. The next two areas of highest participation were employment and education (with slightly less than one-third of inmate parents participating), followed by parenting (11.9%). Some states offer specific prerelease programming services that address topics related to

Table 1. Service Types that Incarcerated Parents Report Would Be Helpful during Prison and after Release from Prison in Terms of Parenting Their Children.

During prison	n	%
Parent skills training	207	57.7
Individual and interpersonal skills	133	37.0
Contact opportunities with family/caregivers	77	21.5
Substance abuse/mental health treatment	71	19.8
Employment/education training	57	15.9
Social support	17	4.7
Religion/spirituality	11	3.1
Housing stability	11	3.1
After release		
Employment/education training	161	44.9
Individual and interpersonal skills training	147	40.9
Parenting skills training	98	27.3
Substance abuse/mental health treatment	74	20.6
Contact/relationships with family/caregivers	65	18.1
Housing stability	62	17.3
Social support	57	15.9
Parole	23	6.4
Religion/spirituality	15	4.2

housing, life skills, and childcare/custody, however, only one-third of incarcerated parents received this type of service.

Once released, formerly incarcerated parents may receive short-term, multiservice residential services, transitional services, reentry programming, or additional assistance through community programs. The participation rate in these types of programs is unknown. Unfortunately, the research on the effectiveness of these types of programs for formerly incarcerated individuals is limited.

Community context

The challenges faced within the home are compounded by the risks the families can face at the community level, including criminal exposure, high neighborhood unemployment and poverty, substandard housing, and poor-quality schools and support services. Research has demonstrated not only the deleterious effects that communities of concentrated disadvantage can have on child development but also that clinical and other remedial types of interventions are likely to be insufficient to promote widespread and long-term change (Dalton, Elias, & Wandersman, 2001; Rappaport, 1977). This idea has been discussed at the national level since the 1950s and recently has been supported in a National Research Council and Institute of Medicine report (2009), which stressed the importance and, perhaps necessity, of multicomponent and multilevel (e.g., child, family, and community) preventive approaches to promote positive development among children. In working with children of incarcerated parents, comprehensive community-based approaches are likely to be especially important given the number and different types of risks that may come into play.

Intervening at the community level is not a new idea. In fact, during the past three decades, comprehensive community initiatives have become an increasingly popular development strategy for communities of concentrated disadvantage (Messinger, 2004). For example, in the early 1990s, Communities that Care, a prevention "operating system," was introduced as a way to help support communities in implementing a community prevention initiative (Hawkins & Catalano, 1992). The recent interest of the federal government in neighborhood revitalization and community initiatives —through such efforts as the Department of Education's Promise Neighborhood Initiative, the Department of Justice's Byrne Criminal Justice Innovation program, and the Department of Housing and Urban Development's Choice Neighborhood—has provided a boost to the idea of comprehensive community efforts in action around the country. The underlying idea in all these efforts is that communities work together across systems to assess the strengths and needs within the community and strategize ways to develop, implement, and/or connect multiple interventions at different intervention levels (i.e., community, organizational, programmatic). Supporters of comprehensive initiatives argue that this method is one of the best ways to address interrelated and concentrated community level problems (e.g., criminality, violence, unemployment, poverty) (Cadora, Swartz, & Gorden, 2003; Ewalt, 1997; Rothman & Zald, 1995).

Of all the interventions focused on supporting children of incarcerated parents and their families, this level of intervention is the least developed or examined. However, based on the identified needs of children and families impacted by incarceration, some helpful community-level interventions could include such activities as: the development of a comprehensive and coordinated system of care to attend to the needs of the children and families impacted by incarceration; an expansion of economic opportunities and social capital within a community of concentrated disadvantage; increased availability and access to reentry programs; and transitional and permanent housing for formerly incarcerated parents and their families. Focusing prevention efforts on communities of concentrated disadvantage to mitigate these community-level challenges might be a way to efficiently and effectively make a difference for a large number of children of incarcerated parents and their families.

Toward building a multilevel prevention strategy to support children

Research on specific interventions for children of incarcerated parents and their families is just beginning to emerge, making now an ideal time to start conceptualizing how a complementary set of interventions might be combined to create an effective, comprehensive prevention strategy to address the complexity and multilevel nature of the issue. Developing, launching, and sustaining such a multilevel prevention strategy are likely to be challenging. This is true when addressing any public health issue, but it may be especially true for a strategy targeting a population that can be difficult to engage for long periods of time, facing multiple contextual challenges, and with frequent fluctuations in roles, relationships, and residences (Bank, Reddick, Weeber, & Swineheart, 2004; Eddy et al., 2008; Eddy, Powell, Szubka, McCool, & Kuntz, 2001).

There are models available that could guide the work ahead. For example, Komro, Flay, and Biglan (2011) introduced the Creating Nurturing Environments model, a developmentally informed, science-based model to help guide comprehensive efforts to promote positive youth development within communities of concentrated disadvantage (see Figure 1). Informed by Brofenbrenner's Ecological Theory (1986), the framework summarizes potent malleable influences within children's environments (e.g., family, schools, community) that can help promote optimal child development in the areas of cognitive development, social/emotional/behavioral competence, and psychological/physical health. With an eye toward balancing comprehensiveness and parsimony, the model focuses on three key proximal influences

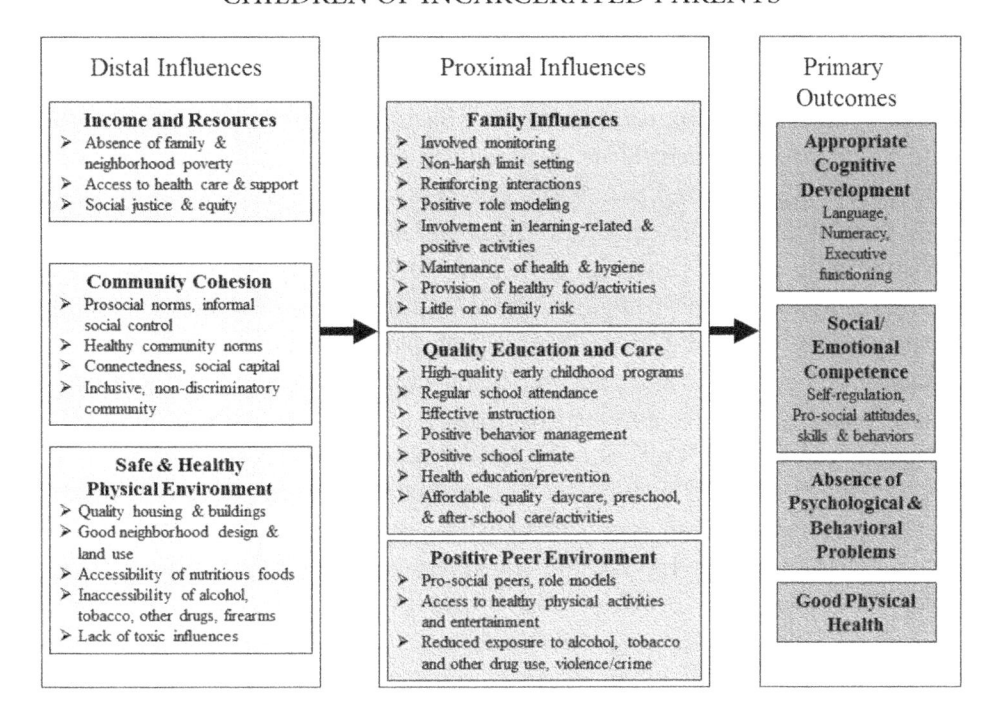

Distal Influences	Proximal Influences	Primary Outcomes
Income and Resources ➤ Absence of family & neighborhood poverty ➤ Access to health care & support ➤ Social justice & equity	**Family Influences** ➤ Involved monitoring ➤ Non-harsh limit setting ➤ Reinforcing interactions ➤ Positive role modeling ➤ Involvement in learning-related & positive activities ➤ Maintenance of health & hygiene ➤ Provision of healthy food/activities ➤ Little or no family risk	**Appropriate Cognitive Development** Language, Numeracy, Executive functioning
Community Cohesion ➤ Prosocial norms, informal social control ➤ Healthy community norms ➤ Connectedness, social capital ➤ Inclusive, non-discriminatory community	**Quality Education and Care** ➤ High-quality early childhood programs ➤ Regular school attendance ➤ Effective instruction ➤ Positive behavior management ➤ Positive school climate ➤ Health education/prevention ➤ Affordable quality daycare, preschool, & after-school care/activities	**Social/Emotional Competence** Self-regulation, Pro-social attitudes, skills & behaviors
Safe & Healthy Physical Environment ➤ Quality housing & buildings ➤ Good neighborhood design & land use ➤ Accessibility of nutritious foods ➤ Inaccessibility of alcohol, tobacco, other drugs, firearms ➤ Lack of toxic influences	**Positive Peer Environment** ➤ Pro-social peers, role models ➤ Access to healthy physical activities and entertainment ➤ Reduced exposure to alcohol, tobacco and other drug use, violence/crime	**Absence of Psychological & Behavioral Problems** **Good Physical Health**

Figure 1. Theoretical model of child adjustment. From Komro et al. (2011).

(i.e., family, daycare/school, and peers) and three key distal influences (i.e., income and resources, social cohesion/capital, and the physical environment within the community) that research has found to affect child development.

As suggested in the model, a child's family can influence the development of the child in numerous ways (i.e., positive parenting practices, modeling prosocial behaviors, minimizing family risk) and, as such, can have an important effect on child development, especially when the children are young. Likewise, quality daycare and schools can increase the likelihood that children develop healthy cognitive, socioemotional, and behavioral skills by using quality educational practices and creating a positive, nurturing environment. The peer environment becomes increasingly important during the adolescent years, when friends may influence and reinforce decisions and behaviors to a high degree. Having prosocial relationships, and engaging in positive interactions and activities with peers can help youth develop into healthy, prosocial adults.

In terms of distal influences, an individual's access to income and resources play a major part in a child's development. Poverty can decrease access to important resources (i.e., food, housing, educational opportunities, and dental, psychological, and health care, educational opportunities), increase family stress and conflict, and expose the individual to harmful influences (i.e., violence, toxins). Social cohesion and social capital within a community can help support and foster healthy prosocial norms and relationships, social inclusion, and access to resources and opportunities for children and families alike. Finally, the physical environment (i.e., decayed/abandoned buildings, physical disorder, substandard housing) can impair a child's development directly or indirectly through the impact on proximal influences (e.g., decreased social cohesion, an increase in crime and injuries).

By identifying key proximal and distal influences, the Creating Nurturing Environments model provides a helpful backdrop for conceptualizing a multilevel approach to strengthen those environments that are positive in the development of children of incarcerated parents while lessening harmful influences. This holistic and comprehensive conceptualization of a strategy is vital to building effective and lasting changes to advance the health and well-being of children and families impacted by parental incarceration.

With this framework in mind, it is clear that there is considerable work to be done to develop such a comprehensive prevention strategy for children and families impacted by parental incarceration. As a first step, the field needs to continue to develop, adapt, and evaluate specific interventions focused on key proximal and distal influences that are particularly relevant to children and families impacted by parental incarceration. While there has been a rapid rise in the development and implementation of programs to support the children of incarcerated parents and their families, these programs are still fairly scarce and limited in scope across the United States. Efforts need to continue to focus on developing and/or adapting interventions, especially in those domains where there are currently few interventions (i.e., schools, peers, and communities). As interventions are implemented, rigorously evaluating the efficacy and effectiveness of these interventions, and the moderators and mediators of program impacts, will be critical to understanding when, how, and for whom they should be used.

As promising interventions are identified, research will be needed on how to best combine interventions across different contextual levels to address the multiple challenges that children and families face. Given the immense variation that can exist between criminal justice–involved families and the communities that surround them, having a tailored approach is likely to be essential. To do this well will require thoroughly assessing the environments surrounding a particular child, including their families, schools, and peers, as well as their broader community.

Such an assessment would serve as an entree into a tailored, multilevel prevention strategy which brings together appropriate interventions to address the strengths, needs, and priorities relevant to a specific child and family, but to other children and families within their community. A tailored, multilevel prevention strategy focused on a certain child or family might combine such interventions as child mentoring, a parenting course, and community referrals to address specific challenges faced by the family (e.g., employment, housing, substance abuse, interpersonal issues), while simultaneously developing a formalized, comprehensive, and coordinated response among service providers within a community to attend to the different potential challenges facing children and families with an incarcerated parent.

Interest in and support for such multimodal, multilevel efforts for families impacted by parental incarceration are beginning to emerge. For example, the Administration for Children and Families recently introduced the Responsible Fatherhood Opportunities for Reentry and Mobility (ReFORM) initiative (2015). Five demonstration projects across the United States (in Kentucky, New York, Ohio, Washington State, and West Virginia) are currently exploring ways to integrate community-centered, skill-based support services for fathers reentering into the community. Each project combines multiple interventions to address three main issues: economic stability, parenting, and healthy relationships. For instance, Washington State's project, The Pre- and Post-Release Multimodal Intervention for Incarcerated Fathers (Becker-Green, House-Higgins, Eddy, Kjellstrand, Harris, Harding, & Meinko, 2015), integrates ongoing case management with a set of evidence-based and promising programs (including Parenting Inside Out: Eddy et al., 2008; The Seven Principles for Making a Marriage Work: Gottman & Silver, 2015; Walking the Line: Markman, Stanley, & Blumberg, 2010; Job Seeking Skills: Washington State Employment Security Department, 2010) to address core needs of incarcerated fathers before and after release from prison. Beginning up to 9 months before release and lasting 9 months after release, the program will provide eligible fathers with direct support and training that are responsive to individual strengths, needs, personal history, and family dynamics. At the community level, case managers will work within local counties to align additional resources and supports for the fathers, their children, and their families to ease the transition of the father back into the community and family. Critical in these demonstration projects will be to carefully document, share, and disseminate key findings related to program development, implementation, overall impact, and lessons learned. Doing so can help accelerate the development, improvement, and uptake of interventions and strategies that are so sorely needed for these children, parents, and families.

Conclusion

With an increasing amount of research demonstrating the harmful effects of parental incarceration on children, families, and communities, attention is needed from the research, practice, and policy communities on developing effective interventions to mitigate these unintended consequences of parental incarceration. This article summarized some of the common risks facing children of incarcerated parents as well as existing interventions designed to help support children and families overcome these challenges. Individually, each risk can be detrimental to a child's development; combined, the harm can be multiplied. The variability and multilevel nature of the risks associated with parental incarceration highlight the difficulty in finding solutions. With the number of issues that come into play, it is clear that an intervention strategy is needed that can both address the common challenges facing families across contextual levels, but also can be tailored to accommodate the unique situations of each child, parent, and family.

With research on the effectiveness of interventions beginning to emerge, now is an ideal time to conceptualize how to best combine different interventions to create an effective, comprehensive prevention strategy to address the complexity and multilevel nature of the issue. The potential directions suggested in this article can help the field move forward toward creating such a tailored, multilevel prevention strategy to help support children of incarcerated parents. Such a strategy is critical for promoting effective, positive, and lasting changes in the health, well-being, and future of millions of children, families, and communities left struggling in the wake of mass incarceration.

References

Ackerman, B. P., Brown, E. D., & Izard, C. E. (2004). The relations between contextual risk, earned income, and the school adjustment of children from economically disadvantaged families. *Developmental Psychology, 40*(2), 204–216. doi:10.1037/0012-1649.40.2.204

Arditti, J. A. (2012). Child trauma within the context of parental incarceration: A family process perspective. *Journal of Family Theory & Review, 4*(3), 181–219. doi:10.1111/j.1756-2589.2012.00128.x

Aseltine, R. H., Jr., Dupre, M., & Lamlein, P. (2000). Mentoring as a drug prevention strategy: An evaluation of across ages. *Adolescent & Family Health, 1*(1), 11–20.

Bales, W., & Mears, D. (2008). Inmate social ties and the transition to society: Does visitation reduce recidivism? *Journal of Research in Crime and Delinquency, 45*(3), 287–321. doi:10.1177/0022427808317574

Bank, L., Reddick, C., Weeber, G., & Swineheart, A. (2004). Motivation and parenting with an offender population. *Community Corrections Report on Law and Corrections Practice, 11*(4), 37–38.

Baumer, E. P., O'Donnell, I., & Hughes, N. (2009). The porous prison: A note on the rehabilitative potential of visits home. *The Prison Journal, 89*(1), 119. doi:10.1177/0032885508330430

Becker-Green, J., House-Higgins, C., Eddy, J. M., Kjellstrand, J. M., Harris, M., Harding, M., & Meiko, J. (2015). *A pre- and post-release multimodal intervention for incarcerated fathers targeting parenting, economic stability, and healthy relationships*. Funded grant received by Washington State Department of Corrections from the U.S. Administration for Children and Families.

Bronfenbrenner, U. (1986). Ecology of the family as a context for human development: Research perspectives. *Developmental Psychology, 22*(6), 723–742. doi:10.1037/0012-1649.22.6.723

Byrne, M., Goshin, L., & Joestl, S. (2010). Intergenerational transmission of attachment for infants raised in a prison nursery. *Attachment & Human Development, 12*(4), 375–393. doi:10.1080/14616730903417011

Cadora, E., Swartz, C., & Gordon, M. (2003). Criminal justice and health and human services: An exploration of overlapping needs, resources, and interests in Brooklyn neighborhoods. In J. Travis, & M. Waul (Eds.), *Prisoners once removed: The impact of incarceration and reentry on children, families, and communities* (pp. 285–311). Washington, DC: Urban Institute Press.

Cho, R. M. (2010). Maternal incarceration and children's adolescent outcomes: Timing and dosage. *Social Service Review, 84*(2), 257–282. doi:10.1086/653456

Clement, M. J. (1993). Parenting in prison: A national survey of programs for incarcerated women. *Journal of Offender Rehabilitation, 19*(1–2), 89–100. doi:10.1300/J076v19n01_06

Connell, A. M., & Goodman, S. H. (2002). The association between psychopathology in fathers versus mothers and children's internalizing and externalizing behavior problems: A meta-analysis. *Psychological Bulletin, 128*(5), 746–773. doi:10.1037/0033-2909.128.5.746

Dalton, J. H., Elias, M. J., & Wandersman, A. (2001). *Community psychology: Linking individuals and communities*. Belmont, CA, US: Wadsworth/Thomson Learning.

DuBois, D. L., Holloway, B. E., Valentine, J. C., & Cooper, H. (2002). Effectiveness of mentoring programs for youth: A meta-analytic review. *American Journal of Community Psychology, 30*(2), 157–197. doi:10.1023/A:1014628810714

Eddy, B. A., Powell, M. J., Szubka, M. H., McCool, M. L., & Kuntz, S. (2001). Challenges in research with incarcerated parents and importance in violence prevention. *American Journal of Preventive Medicine, 20*(1, Supplement 1), 56–62. doi:10.1016/S0749-3797%2800%2900273-7

Eddy, J. M. (2014). *Parent Child Study* (Unpublished data). Oregon Social Learning Center, Eugene, OR.

Eddy, J. M., Cearley, J. J., Bergen, J., & Stern-Carusone, J. (2013). Children of incarcerated parents. In D. L. DuBois & M. Karcher (Eds.), *Handbook of youth mentoring* (2nd ed.). Thousand Oaks, CA: Sage.

Eddy, J. M., Kjellstrand, J. M., Martinez, C. R., Jr., & Newton, R. (2010). Theory-based multimodal parenting intervention for incarcerated parents and their families. In J. M. Eddy, & J. Pochlmann (Eds.), *Children of incarcerated parents: Multidisciplinary perspectives on research, intervention, and policy* (pp. 237–261). Washington, DC: Urban Institute Press.

Eddy, J. M., Martinez, C. R., Jr., & Burraston, B. (2013). A randomized controlled trial of a parent management training program for incarcerated parents: Proximal impacts. In J. Poehlmann & J. M. Eddy (Eds.), Relationship processes and resilience in children with incarcerated parents. *Monographs of the Society for Research in Child Development, 78*(3), 75–93. doi:10.1111/mono.12022

Eddy, J. M., Martinez, C. R., Jr., Schiffmann, T., Newton, R., Olin, L., Leve, L. . . . Shortt, J. W. (2008). Development of a multisystemic parent management training intervention for incarcerated parents, their children and families. *Clinical Psychologist, 12*(3), 86–98. doi:10.1080/13284200802495461

Eddy, J. M., & Poehlmann, J. (Eds.). (2010). *Children of incarcerated parents: A handbook for researchers and practitioners*. Washington, DC: Urban Institute Press.

Ewalt, P. L. (1997). The revitalization of impoverished communities. *Social Work, 42*(5), 413–414. doi:10.1093/sw/42.5.413

Foster, H. (2011). Incarcerated parents and health: Investigating role inoccupancy strains by gender. *Women & Criminal Justice, 21*(3), 225–249. doi:10.1080/08974454.2011.584463

Gaes, G. G., & Kendig, N. (2003). The skills sets and health care needs of released offenders. In J. Travis, & M. Waul (Eds.), *Prisoners once removed: The impact of incarceration and reentry on children, families, and communities*. Washington, DC: Urban Institute Press.

Glaze, L. E., & Maruschak, L. M. (2008). *Parents in prison and their minor children*. Washington, DC: US Department of Justice, Office of Justice Programs.

Gonzalez, P., Romero, T., & Cerbana, C. B. (2007). Parent education program for incarcerated mothers in Colorado. *Journal of Correctional Education, 58*(4), 357–373.

Gottman, J. M., & Silver, N. (2015). *The seven principles for making marriage work: A practical guide from the country's foremost relationship expert* (2nd ed.). New York, NY: Harmony Books.

Gutman, L. M., Sameroff, A. J., & Cole, R. (2003). Academic growth curve trajectories from 1st grade to 12th grade: Effects of multiple social risk factors and preschool child factors. *Developmental Psychology, 39*(4), 777–790. doi:10.1037/0012-1649.39.4.777

Hairston, C. F. (2007). *Focus on children with incarcerated parents: An overview of the research literature*. Baltimore, MD: Annie E. Casey Foundation.

Hawkins, J. D., & Catalano, R. F. (1992). *Communities that care: Action for drug abuse prevention*. San Francisco, CA: Jossey-Bass, Inc.

Johnston, D. (1995). Parent-child visits in jails. *Children's Environments, 12*(1), 25–38. http://www.jstor.org/stable/41514962

Kjellstrand, J. M., & Eddy, J. (2011). Parental incarceration during childhood, family context, and youth problem behavior across adolescence. *Journal of Offender Rehabilitation, 50*(1), 18–36. doi:10.1080/10509674.2011.536720

Klaw, E. L., Rhodes, J. E., & Fitzgerald, L. F. (2003). Natural mentors in the lives of African American adolescent mothers: Tracking relationships over time. *Journal of Youth and Adolescence, 32*(3), 223–232. doi:10.1023/A:1022551721565

Komro, K. A., Flay, B. R., & Biglan, A. (2011). Creating nurturing environments: A science-based framework for promoting child health and development within high-poverty neighborhoods. *Clinical Child and Family Psychology Review, 14*(2), 111–134. doi:10.1007/s10567-011-0095-2

La Vigne, N. G., Naser, R. L., Brooks, L. E., & Castro, J. L. (2005). Examining the effect of incarceration and in-prison family contact on prisoners' family relationships. *Journal of Contemporary Criminal Justice, 21*(4), 314–335. doi:10.1177/1043986205281727

Laakso, J., & Nygaard, J. (2012). Children of incarcerated parents: How a mentoring program can make a difference. *Social Work in Public Health, 27*(1–2), 12–28. doi:10.1080/19371918.2012.629892

Lipsey, M. W., & Derzon, J. H. (1998). Predictors of violent or serious delinquency in adolescence and early adulthood: A synthesis of longitudinal research. In R. Loeber, & D. P. Farrington (Eds.), *Serious and violent juvenile offenders: Risk factors and successful interventions* (pp. 86–105). Thousand Oaks, CA: Sage Publications.

Loper, A. B., & Novero, C. (2010). Parenting programs for prisoners: Current research and new directions. In J. Poehlmann & M. Eddy (Eds.), *Children of incarcerated parents: A handbook for researchers and practitioners* (pp. 189–216). Washington, DC: Urban Institute Press.

Loper, A. B., & Tuerk, E. H. (2011). Improving the emotional adjustment and communication patterns of incarcerated mothers: Effectiveness of a prison parenting intervention. *Journal of Child and Family Studies, 20*(1), 89–101. doi:10.1007/s10826-010-9381-8

LoSciuto, L., Rajala, A. K., Townsend, T. N., & Taylor, A. S. (1996). An outcome evaluation of across ages: An intergenerational mentoring approach to drug prevention. *Journal of Adolescent Research, 11*(1), 116–129. doi:10.1177/0743554896111007

Markman, H. J., Stanley, S. M., & Blumberg, S. L. (2010). *Fighting for your marriage*. San Francisco, CA: Jossey-Bass.

Maruschak, L. M., & Mumola, C. J. (2010). Incarcerated parents and their children: Findings from the Bureau of Justice Statistics. In J. M. Eddy, & J. Poehlmann (Eds.), *Children of incarcerated parents: A handbook for researchers and practitioners* (pp. 33–54). Washington, DC: Urban Institute Press.

Masten, A. S., & Coatsworth, J. (1998). The development of competence in favorable and unfavorable environments: Lessons from research on successful children. *American Psychologist, 53*(2), 205–220. doi:10.1037/0003-066X.53.2.205

Messinger, L. (2004). Comprehensive community initiatives: A rural perspective. *Social Work, 49*(4), 535–546. doi:10.1093/sw/49.4.535

Miller, A. L., Weston, L. E., Perryman, J., Horwitz, T., Franzen, S., & Cochran, S. (2014). Parenting while incarcerated: Tailoring the strengthening families program for use with jailed mothers. *Children and Youth Services Review, 44*, 163–170. doi:10.1016/j.childyouth.2014.06.013

National Research Council and Institute of Medicine. (2009). *Preventing mental, emotional, and behavioral disorders among young people: Progress and possibilities. Committee on prevention of mental disorders and substance abuse among children, youth, and young adults: Research advances and promising interventions.* Washington, DC: The National Academies Press.

Nelson, M., & Trone, J. (2000). *Why planning for release matters.* New York, NY: Vera Institute of Justice. Retrieved March 31, 2016, from http://www.vera.org/sites/default/files/resources/downloads/IIB_planning_for_release.pdf

Nichols, E. B., & Loper, A. B. (2012). Incarceration in the household: Academic outcomes of adolescents with an incarcerated household member. *Journal of Youth and Adolescence, 41*(11), 1455–1471. doi:10.1007/s10964-012-9780-9

Parke, R. D., & Clarke-Stewart, K. A. (2001). *Effects of parental incarceration on young children.* Washington, DC: U.S. Department of Health and Human Services.

Phillips, S. D., Gleeson, J. P., & Waites-Garrett, M. (2009). Substance-abusing parents in the criminal justice system: Does substance abuse treatment improve their children's outcomes? *Journal of Offender Rehabilitation, 48*(2), 120–138. doi:10.1080/10509670802640925

Phillips, S. D., & O'Brien, P. (2012). Learning from the Ground Up: Responding to children affected by parental incarceration. *Social Work in Public Health, 27*(1-2), 29–44. doi:10.1080/19371918.2012.629914

Pizzarro, J. M., Stenius, V. M. K., & Pratt, T. C. (2006). Myths, realities, and the politics of punishment in American society. *Criminal Justice Policy Review, 17*(1), 6–21. doi:10.1177/0887403405275015

Poehlmann, J., Dallaire, D., Loper, A. B., & Shear, L. D. (2010). Children's contact with their incarcerated parents: Research findings and recommendations. *American Psychologist 65, 65*(6), 575–598. doi:10.1037/a0020279

Rappaport, J. (1977). *Community psychology: Values, research, and action.* New York, NY: Holt, Rinehart & Winston.

Reid, J. B., Patterson, G. R., & Snyder, J. J. (2002). *Antisocial behavior in children and adolescents: A developmental analysis and model for intervention.* Washington, DC: American Psychological Association.

Rishel, C., Sales, E., & Koeske, G. F. (2005). Relationships with non-parental adults and child behavior. *Child & Adolescent Social Work Journal, 22*(1), 19–34. doi:10.1007/s10560-005-2546-4

Rothman, J., & Zald, M. N. (1995). *Planning and policy practice* (5th ed.). Itasco, IL: F.E. Peacock.

Sevigny, E. L., Fuleihan, B. K., & Ferdik, F. V. (2013). Do drug courts reduce the use of incarceration?: A meta-analysis. *Journal of Criminal Justice, 41*(6), 416–425. doi:10.1016/j.jcrimjus.2013.06.005

Shlafer, R. J., Poehlmann, J., Coffino, B., & Hanneman, A. (2009). Mentoring children with incarcerated parents: Implications for research, practice, and policy. *Family Relations, 58* (5), 507–519. doi:10.1111/fare.2009.58.issue-5

Springer, D. W., Lynch, C., & Rubin, A. (2000). Effects of a solution-focused mutual aid group for Hispanic children of incarcerated parents. *Child & Adolescent Social Work Journal, 17*(6), 431–442. doi:10.1023/A:1026479727159

Travis, J., Waul, M., & Geraghty, T. F. (2004). Prisoners once removed: The impact of incarceration and reentry on children, families, and communities. *Journal of Criminal Law and Criminology, 94*(4), 1149–1162.

Turanovic, J. J., Rodriguez, N., & Pratt, T. C. (2012). The collateral consequences of incarceration revisited: A qualitative analysis of the effects on caregivers of children of incarcerated parents. *Criminology: An Interdisciplinary Journal, 50*(4), 913–959. doi:10.1111/j.1745-9125.2012.00283.x

Wachs, T. D. (1996). Known and potential processes underlying developmental trajectories in childhood and adolescence. *Developmental Psychology, 32*(4), 796–801. doi:10.1037/0012-1649.32.4.796

Washington State Employment Security Department. (2010). *Job seeking skills.* Retrieved from https://www.pdffiller.com/en/project/63270004.htm?form_id=233073101

Weissman, M., & LaRue, C. M. (1998). Earning trust from youths with none to spare. *Child Welfare: Journal of Policy, Practice, and Program, 77*(5), 579–594.

Werner, E. E. (1989). High-Risk Children in Young Adulthood: A Longitudinal Study from Birth to 32 Years. *American Journal of Orthopsychiatry, 59*(1), 72–81. doi:10.1111/j.1939-0025.1989.tb01636.x

Western, B., & Wildeman, C. (2009). The black family and mass incarceration. *The ANNALS of the American Academy of Political and Social Science, 621*(1), 221–242. doi:10.1177/0002716208324850

Zwiebach, L., Rhodes, J. E., & Dun Rappaport, C. (2010). Mentoring interventions for children of incarcerated parents. In J. M. Eddy, & J. Poehlmann (Eds.), *Children of incarcerated parents* (pp. 217–236). Washington, DC: The Urban Institute Press.

Index

Note: **Bold face** page numbers refer to tables & *italic* page numbers refer to figures.

A
AAI *see* Adult Attachment Interview
Administration for Children and Families 123
adolescence: as sensitive period 44; substance abuse 43–4
Adoption and Safe Families Act of 1997 (ASFA) 36
Adult Attachment Interview (AAI) 29; classification 32, **32**; research questions 30–1; results/outcomes 34
Adult Static Risk Assessment (ASRA) 83
"adverse childhood experience" 1
African Americans, ethnic/racial disparity 60, 62, **66**–7, 68
Aguiar, Chyla M. 2
alcohol use: binge drinking 46; early initiation of 45–6; treatment for 47–8
American Indians, ethnic/racial disparity 60, **66**–7, 68
analyses of variance (ANOVAs) 65
area under the curve (AUC) statistic 86
ASFA *see* Adoption and Safe Families Act of 1997
ASRA *see* Adult Static Risk Assessment
attachment theory 5, 29
AUC statistic *see* area under the curve statistic

B
Bedford Hills Correctional Facility for Women 1
"best interests" of child 79
Bick, Esther 5
binge drinking 46
BJS *see* Bureau of Justice Statistics
Borja, Sharon 2
Bowlby, John 5
Bowlby's theory of attachment 29
Brofenbrenner's Ecological Theory 120
Bureau of Justice Statistics (BJS) 42
Burraston, Bert O. 2
Byrne Criminal Justice Innovation program 119

C
caregivers: grandmothers 26, 35; multiple 13; and relational health 18
CCOs *see* community corrections officers
chemical dependency 7
child adjustment 116; individual therapy 116–17; mentoring 116; support groups 117; theoretical model of *121*
childhood victimization 60, 61
Children's Administration, Washington 79
child welfare system: infants' experiences in 20; involvement 60
chi-square tests 65
Choice Neighborhood 119
'Communities that Care' 119
community-based sentencing 115
community corrections officers (CCOs) 79, 81, 89
Community Parenting Alternative (CPA) **81**, 82–3
comprehensive community initiatives 119–20
Condon, Marie-Celeste 1
CPA *see* Community Parenting Alternative
Creating Nurturing Environments model 120, 122
criminal behavior 96

INDEX

D
Davis, Laurel 2
DEL *see* Department of Early Learning
Department of Corrections (DOC) 63, 79, 80, 98
Department of Early Learning (DEL) 80
Department of Justice's recidivism report 94
Diagnostic and Statistical Manual of Mental Disorders, Fourth Edition (DSM-4) criteria 46–7; for substance abuse/dependence 47
disorganized-disoriented attachment 28, 35
drug offenses 27
drug use 52; treatment for 47–8; *see also* alcohol use
DSM-4 criteria *see Diagnostic and Statistical Manual of Mental Disorders, Fourth Edition* criteria

E
Early Head Start (EHS) program 6, 19
early relational health 5 *see also* Residential Parenting Program
Eddy, J. Mark 2
EHM *see* electronic home monitoring
EHS program *see* Early Head Start program
electronic home monitoring (EHM) 79

F
family contact, in prison 102
Family Educational Rights and Privacy Act 45
family-focused intervention programs 113
Family Offender Sentencing Alternative (FOSA) 80–1, **81**
family reunification group: Adult Attachment Interview 29–31, **32**, 34; data collection 30–1; inclusion criteria for 30; participants in 30; TABS t-scores for **33**
Flesch Reading Ease Scale 31
FOSA *see* Family Offender Sentencing Alternative

G
Gina case study 89–90
"good enough" mother 26
grandmothers, as primary caregivers 26, 35

H
Harden, Jones 20
Harris, Marian S. 1
household substance abuse 49
Housing Opportunity Act (1996) 28, 37

I
incarcerated mothers 25–6; Adoption and Safe Families Act (1997) 36; Anti-Drug Abuse Act (1986) 37; clinical treatment for 36; depression 35; drug offenses 27; feelings of pain 35; grandmothers, as primary caregivers 26, 35; Housing Opportunity Act (1996) 28, 37; limitations of study 37; Quality Housing and Work Responsibility Act (1998) 28, 37; reasons for incarceration 27–8; social workers, contact with 36; time concept 36; trauma and attachment issues 28–30, 37; in United States 26–7; *see also* family reunification group
Individual Family Service Plans 7
infant observation 5, 8–9
inmate parents, service types 117–18, **118**
Institute of Medicine report (2009) 113, 119
intergenerational incarceration 62–3
internal working model 32–3
intervention strategies 112; child adjustment 116–17, *121*; community-based sentencing 115; community context 119–20; effectiveness of 124; family context 117–19, **118**; mentoring 116; parenting classes 114; remote contact 114–15; support groups 117; visitation programs 114

J
juvenile felony conviction 86, **87**
juvenile justice system 62

K
Kjellstrand, Jean 2

L
Latinos, ethnic/racial disparity 63, **66–7**, 68
Lazzari, Sarah R. 2
learning problems 101
Leavell, Susan 2
life-course paradigm 95
life histories of incarcerated parents 58–9; African Americans 60, 62, **66–7**, 68; American Indians 60, **66–7**, 68; analyses of variance 65; childhood victimization 60, 61; child welfare involvement 60; chi-square tests 65; eligibility criteria 64; intergenerational incarceration 62–3; juvenile justice involvement 62; Latinos 63, **66–7**, 68; mental health issues 61–2; participants' recruitment 64–5; PIO

INDEX

intervention 63; race and ethnicity **66–7**; substance abuse problems 61–2; trauma exposure 60–1; Whites 60, 61, 64, **66–7**, 68
lifetime marijuana use 46
'living with children' 97
logistic regression models 49, 50, **51**

M
marijuana use 46
mental health: diagnoses 101, 104; issues 61–2; programs 118; of RPP mothers 17
mentoring 116
Miller, Keva M. 2
Minnesota Student Survey (2013) 45
mother-child relationship 25–6
multilevel prevention strategy 113, 120–3
multiple caregivers 13

N
National Research Council report (2009) 113, 119
National Survey of Children's Health 42

O
Offender Needs Assessment (ONA) 83, 84
"one-size-fits-all" approach 112
"One Strike" policy 37
overarching emotion 6

P
parent-child attachments 29, 95–6
Parent Child Study (2013) 63, 98, 117
parent/family intervention programs 113; community-based sentencing 115; parenting classes 114; remote contact 114–15; visitation programs 114
parenting classes 114
Parenting Inside Out (PIO) program 97; age and gender 101; analytic strategy 102; control conditions 99–100; descriptive statistics **100**; hypotheses 97–8; interaction variable 101; living with children 97, 101; mental health/learning problems 101; participants' eligibility criteria 98; participants in intervention 99, 105–6; postrelease arrests 100; preventive intervention strategy 105–6; prior arrests 101; racial and ethnic study 63; randomization 98–9; releasing institutions 98; results, analysis of 102–4; time in prison 101; Zero-Inflated Negative Binomial Regression model 102, **103**

Parenting Sentencing Alternative (PSA): Adult Static Risk Assessment 83; area under the curve statistic 86; Community Parenting Alternative **81**, 82–3; comparison group development 85–6; control variables 84; dependent variable 84; development 79–80; eligibility and implementation 80; Family Offender Sentencing Alternative 80–1, **81**; felony recidivism 86, **87**; Gina case study 89–90; independent variable 84; limitations of 87–8; propensity score match 84–6, **85**; research question 83; Washington State Legislature 78
parent management training (PMT) 96–7
partner violence 61
Pathfinders of Oregon 98
physical violence 61
PIO program see Parenting Inside Out program
PMT see parent management training
postrelease arrests 100, 104, *104*
Pre- and Post-Release Multimodal Intervention for Incarcerated Fathers 123
prescription drugs, recreational use of 46
prior arrests 101, 104, *104*
prison nurseries 115
Promise Neighborhood Initiative 119
Protection of Pupil Rights Amendment 45
PSA see Parenting Sentencing Alternative
psychic trauma 28

Q
quality daycare and schools 121
Quality Housing and Work Responsibility Act (1998) 28, 37

R
race and ethnicity: disparities 62; in life histories of incarcerated parents **66–7**; PIO intervention 63; substance abuse 48–9
RAR see Risk Assessment Report
recidivism: Department of Justice's report on 94; factors associated with 95; Parenting Sentencing Alternative study 84, 86, **87**, 88
reentering society 78; issues regarding reentry 94–5; theoretical foundations 95–7; see also Parenting Inside Out program
reflective capacity 13

INDEX

ReFORM initiative *see* Responsible Fatherhood Opportunities for Reentry and Mobility initiative
relational health 5, 6, 12; *see also* Residential Parenting Program
remote contact 114–15
Residential Parenting Program (RPP) 6; bias and trustworthiness 11; consultation model 20; correctional facility 7; empirical phenomenological techniques 9; infant observation 5, 8–9; infants' experiences 10; limitations of 19; local EHS program 7; multiple caregivers 13; offenders in 7–8; overall well-being 11–12, 20; participants in 6–7; Penny and Tommy case 13, 15; positive aspects of 8; reflective capacity 13; relational health 12; research questions 9; second-order constructs 10; unintended effects on participants 10–11; *see also* variability in relational health
Responsible Fatherhood Opportunities for Reentry and Mobility (ReFORM) initiative 123
retraumatization/revictimization 61
Risk Assessment Report (RAR) 80–1
RPP *see* Residential Parenting Program

S
sentencing alternatives 77
Shlafer, Rebecca J. 2
SLT *see* social interaction learning theory
social attachments 95
social bond theory 95
social control theory 95
social interaction learning theory (SLT) 96
STATA statistical software 102
"strengthening families" model 80
STRONG risk assessment 83
substance abuse 2, 42; academic outcomes 52; adolescence, as sensitive period 44; adolescents' environmental exposures 52; adult household 49; age and gender 48; among incarcerated parents 42–3; binge drinking 46; dependent variables 45; descriptive statistics 50, **50**; DSM-4 criteria for 46–7; early alcohol initiation 45–6; genetic risk 52; independent variables 48–9; lifetime marijuana use 46; logistic regression models 49, 50, **51**; Minnesota Student Survey (2013) 45;
missing data, level of 49; parental incarceration and 48, 52; poverty status 48; prescription drugs, recreational use of 46; problems 61–2; race and ethnicity 48–9; recent alcohol use 46; research questions 44, 47; tobacco use 46; urbanicity 49; in youth 43–4
substance dependence, DSM-4 criteria for 47
Substitute Senate Bill 6639 78

T
TABS *see* Trauma Attachment and Belief Scale
time in prison 101
tobacco use 46
total post release arrests *104*
trauma 28, 35; adult exposure to 60–1; and attachment issues 28–30, 37; childhood exposure to 60; complex 35; unresolved issues of 35
Trauma Attachment and Belief Scale (TABS) 30–1; for family reunification group **33**; interpretive range **33**

U
United States: demonstration projects 123; incarceration rate in 58, 93, 111; infants in 4; prisons in 1, 94

V
variability in relational health **14**, 15–16; caregivers' contributions 18; infants' contributions 16; mothers' contributions 16–18, **17**; system-level contributions 18–19
victimization, high rates of 60, 61
violence 43, 59; partner 61
visitation programs 114

W
"war on drugs" 27, 77
Whites, ethnic/racial disparity 60, 61, 64, **66–7**, 68

Z
Zero-Inflated Negative Binomial Regression (ZINB) model 102, **103**
"zero tolerance" policies 27
ZINB model *see* Zero-Inflated Negative Binomial Regression model